HEALTHY HABITS

20 SIMPLE WAYS TO IMPROVE YOUR HEALTH

DAVID & ANNE FRÄHM

JEREMY P. TARCHER/PUTNAM
a member of
Penguin Putnam Inc.
New York

Before beginning any new diet, nutrition, or exercise program, consult with a physician, especially if you have a serious medical condition or are taking medication. The author and publisher disclaim responsibility for any adverse effects or unforeseen consequences resulting from the use of the information contained in this book.

Most Tarcher/Putnam books are available at special quantity discounts for bulk purchases for sales promotions, premiums, fundraising, and educational needs. Special books or book excerpts also can be created to fit specific needs. For details, write or telephone Putnam Special Markets, 200 Madison Avenue, New York, NY 10016; (212) 951-8891.

Jeremy P. Tarcher/Putnam
a member of
Penguin Putnam Inc.
200 Madison Avenue
New York, NY 10016
www.penguinputnam.com

First Jeremy P. Tarcher/Putnam Edition 1998
Originally published by Piñon Press, Colorado Springs, CO

Library of Congress Cataloging-in-Publication Data

Frähm, David J.
Healthy habits : 20 simple ways to improve your health / David and Anne Frähm.
p. cm.
Previously published by Piñon Press in 1993.
Includes bibliographical references.
ISBN 0-87477-918-9
1. Health.   2. Nutrition.   3. Self-care, Health.   I. Frähm, Anne E.
II. Title.
RA776.F799   1998   97-46518 CIP
613—dc21

Printed in the United States of America
1   2   3   4   5   6   7   8   9   10

This book is printed on acid-free paper. ∞

CONTENTS

To the Lord of the harvest,
from whom all things come,
including our bodies
and our responsibility to take care of them.
And to all those health professionals
out there in the front lines,
trying to help people learn
the healthy habits of preventative health care.

ACKNOWLEDGMENTS

A big thank you to our editor and friend, Traci Mullins, for opening doors for us into the world of publishing, and for her work of ensuring that our manuscripts have passed muster.

A big thank you also to Susan Pannell, who has helped to swing wide the publicity doors for our writing efforts.

INTRODUCTION

"I'm so sorry," said the doctor, "the bone marrow transplant just didn't work for you. You've still got a lot of cancer growing in your body."

With that, the final nail in my wife's coffin seemed all but secure. For the previous twelve months we'd been caught up in an aggressive battle against breast cancer which, because of a faulty mammogram reading a year earlier, had been allowed to spread unchecked throughout her body. Cancerous tumors had formed on her skull, ribs, sternum, and pelvic bone—one having actually eaten a stress fracture right into her spine.

At first surgery, radiation, and very intense chemotherapy brought promising results. The cancer count went steadily downward. But then, just as predicted from the beginning by our oncologist, the insidious cancer cells became resistant. As the disease rate started to climb once again, our hopes plummeted.

"There's one last thing we can try," he said. "Let's see if you're a candidate for a bone marrow transplant." At thirty-six years of age, and with a heart judged strong enough to withstand the brutal doses of chemotherapy she was about to receive, Anne was admitted to an isolation room in a hospital ward eight hundred miles away from home. There she racked up fifty-two days of vomiting, blistering, bloating, and very nearly dying. As they say, if the cancer doesn't get you, the treatment will.

Well, with the news from the doctor that the transplant had not accomplished the hoped-for objective of wiping out the cancer, all seemed lost. What now? "Go home," the specialists said. "Eat, drink, and be merry. Live every day to its fullest, for we're quite certain that you don't have many of them left." They didn't really say that last part, but they didn't have to. They'd done all that they knew to do, and it didn't work. We could see it in their eyes. Anne was a goner, at least from their point of view.

My wife has never been one to play the helpless victim. Whatever happens to her in life, she wants to know the facts. She has the nose of a bloodhound to find information and the curiosity of a researcher to ask questions. Soon after getting back home, and still weak from having her body nearly destroyed, she began reading up on the link between diet and degenerative disease. We'd heard a bit of information here and there as we were trudging our way through conventional cancer treatments. But now, as she dug deep into the research, she discovered that nutritionists, chiropractors, and a growing number of physicians were in agreement. The culprit behind the skyrocketing rates in the United States of cancer, heart disease, diabetes, osteoporosis, arthritis, and other related breakdowns in the human machine is the standard American diet, otherwise known as SAD. Not only is diet the chief culprit behind the onset of these diseases, but diet is also the best way to reverse them. A changed diet, radically different from the typical high-fat, high-cholesterol, high-protein, high-acid, low-fiber diet that most of us Americans grow up eating.

After consulting a local nutritionist who read the blood tests and designed a nutritional program just for her, Anne began an intense program of cleaning out her body, rejuvenating her liver, and rebuilding her immune system through a vegetarian diet. Five weeks later our oncologist did a bone marrow test as part of his ongoing monitoring of her condition. To his immense surprise, and to ours, no cancer cells were found. To this he added another test for confirmation. Same results.

"Flabbergasted," he said. "I'm completely flabbergasted!

When you got home from the transplant your cancer was growing back rapidly. I thought you were doomed. It's got to be either divine intervention or your diet."

Truth is, we consider it both. Being God-fearing folk, we're thankful that He's seen fit to keep Anne around through the application of a changed diet. As a result, we feel a genuine sense of duty to help others take better care of their own bodies.

As you can imagine, news spread quickly of Anne's successful battle against cancer. People from around the country and even some from overseas somehow got our phone number and began calling. Fellow cancer warriors who were desperate, grasping at straws for help and hope, wanted to know what she had done. Some were even calling from their hospital beds where they'd just been told that they were out of medical options. It became obvious that a book outlining the details of the nutritional program we used was needed. Thus *A Cancer Battle Plan* was born.

Many of the thousands of responses to that book have come from healthy people asking for more help in knowing what to do to avoid degenerative diseases in the first place. As a result of wanting to respond to that need, this book, our second collaborative effort, has emerged. Thank you so much for picking it up. We hope you will find it a valuable resource, better equipping you to take personal responsibility for your health.

For more information, please drop us a note or call. We'd love to hear from you.

Health*Quarters* Ministries
4141 Sinton Road
Colorado Springs, CO 80907
(719) 593-8694

1
TAKE CHARGE

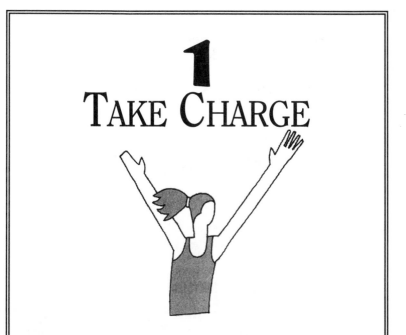

She sneaked in the back door—late to work, eyes brimming with tears, and looking much older than her twenty-something years. She'd been on her way to work when her car stopped dead in its tracks. We gathered around our distraught friend as she began to unfold the details of her story.

"You see, I've never really known much about cars," she confided, wiping away a tear. "I bought Old Blue—that's what I call my car—at this used-car lot. He's been running really great until today. There I was, out in the middle of this huge intersection, when all of a sudden he just quit. I tried and tried to get him started again, but he wouldn't budge. I finally got somebody to come tow him away. The guy at the garage says the engine is frozen up. He said there wasn't a drop of oil left in it. What was I supposed to know about oil? I'd seen some puddles under him now and then, but heck, I didn't know what was going on. I just figured that was part of what normal cars do."

Well, Old Blue never did make it back to the streets again. His engine was completely ruined, and my friend couldn't afford to replace it. She took to riding a bicycle to work, and her car was sold to a junkyard for parts. Every once in a while I'll happen to drive by a car dump and wonder how many other Old Blues are in there that could still be out cruising the highways if their owners had known a little bit about preventative maintenance.

Preventative maintenance, an important concept for all of life. Our cars, our homes, our yards and gardens, and yes, even our bodies—all require it. If you want your car to keep running trouble-free, you're going to have to maintain it. If you want your garden to grow healthy plants, you're going to have to weed and fertilize it. And if you want your body to stay healthy, you're going to have to learn how to feed and take care of it. Good health is not a "freebie"; you have to learn how to cultivate it.

THE STATE OF HEALTH IN THE UNITED STATES TODAY

It is easy to assume that we all want good health. But do we really know all that we need to know in order to keep our bodies in good working condition? Many health-care professionals are warning us today that we Americans are committing slow suicide with our knives and forks around the dinner table.

"Americans don't die, we kill ourselves with our teeth," writes Dr. Gordon Tessler, nutrition consultant and author of *Lazy Person's Guide to Better Nutrition*. "One night, my grandfather went to bed as usual and did not wake up. That is considered a natural death, something which few Americans experience anymore. Instead, most die a premature death which is usually slow, painful and full of great suffering for themselves and their loved ones."[1]

We're all thankful for the advances in sanitation and medicine over the last half century that have brought infectious diseases under control. However, these days Americans are plagued by a whole new set of diseases, unrelated to germs.

"Diet and lifestyle," observes John A. McDougall, medical doctor and author of *McDougall's Medicine*, "are the causes of most of the deaths and disabilities that people suffer in the United States today."[2] Indeed, these are the culprits behind a host of degenerative diseases and their complications which torment our individual and national well-being. They include such maladies as cancer, osteoporosis (loss of bone mass), atherosclerosis (hardening of the arteries), heart attacks, strokes, hypertension (high blood pressure), adult onset diabetes, arthritis, and kidney disease. Of these, heart attacks, cancer, and strokes are the biggest killers.

Heart Attacks

Every year over 1.5 million Americans have heart attacks.[3] They are the leading cause of death in the United States, killing more than 700,000 people annually.[4] As a typical American consuming the typical American diet, your chances of dying from a heart attack at some point in your life are currently about one in two, or 50 percent.[5] In fact, heart attacks and strokes are the leading cause of death and disability in men forty to forty-five years of age.[6]

Cancer

Today in the United States, one out of every three (or 33 percent) of us can expect to develop cancer at some point in our lives. Projections are that by the year 2000, the ratio will be one out of two. And as my oncologist once observed: "They keep coming in here with cancer younger and younger every year." At today's pace, 1.3 million new cancer patients are added to the ranks each year, while another 520,000 see their battle come to an end in death.[7]

Strokes

The third-leading cause of death in the United States is strokes. Every year approximately 550,000 Americans suffer strokes. Of these 162,000 die. Many of those who survive will have lost a great deal of their capacity to live out normal lives.

Scientists estimate that with a few diet and lifestyle changes, 80 percent of the premature (before age sixty-five) deaths and disabilities in our country due to degenerative diseases could be avoided.[8] Many contend that a human body fed and cared for properly has the potential for disease-free health well into the 100-year-old range.[9]

WHY DON'T WE HEAR MORE ABOUT NUTRITION FROM OUR DOCTORS?

The health-care industry in the United States is currently an $800-billion-a-year business. Within the next ten years that figure promises to become $1.2 trillion. Unfortunately, most of this money is spent on repair rather than on prevention. In other words, on treating illness rather than on helping people learn how to stay well. The average doctor receives little, if any, training in preventative medicine. Dr. McDougall notes that "Medical schools have provided a shockingly inadequate education in basic nutrition for doctors. A recent investigation by a Senate subcommittee revealed that the average physician in the United States receives less than 3 hours of training in nutrition during 4 years of medical school and that less than 3% of the licensing exam questions are concerned with nutrition."[10]

In 1985, the president of the American Medical Student Association testified: "Medical education has traditionally focused on the principles of acute episodic health care delivery, overlooking the concepts and application of nutrition and preventative medicine. Nutrition is not well taught, if taught at all, in most medical schools. . . . Because of this deficiency, most physicians-in-training in the United States enter their professional life not equipped with the skills or attitudes to apply nutritional concepts in their practice of medicine."[11]

In other words, the typical medical professional is poorly prepared to help his or her clients effectively cultivate good health and prevent degenerative disorders. "We learned how to use scalpels, deadly drugs, and radiation beams to destroy cancer," observes Stuart Berger, M.D., author of *What Your Doctor Didn't Learn in Medical School*, "but not how the right food and lifestyles could help prevent it in the first place."[12]

A FEW BRIGHT CANDLES IN THE DARK

Admittedly, a growing number of physicians in this country are beginning to practice nutrition as preventative medicine. They are beginning to catch up to the nutritionists, naturopathic physicians, and chiropractors who have been preaching nutrition for years. Many are realizing that not only are diet and healthy habits the key to preventing degenerative disease, but they're also the key to reversing it.

In his book *Dr. Dean Ornish's Program for Reversing Heart Disease*, Dean Ornish, M.D., tells how he became frustrated with what he was being taught in med school concerning treatment for heart patients:

> I saw the limitations of technological approaches (such as coronary bypass surgery) that literally and figuratively "bypassed" the underlying causes of the problem. It was the difference between temporizing and healing. Bypass surgery became, for me, a metaphor for the inadequacy of treating a problem without also addressing the underlying causes. We would operate on patients, their chest pain would usually go away, and they were told that they were cured. Most would go home and continue to do the same things that led to the problem in the first place. They would smoke, eat a high-fat, high cholesterol diet, manage stress poorly, and lead sedentary lives.[13]

In the last several years Dr. Ornish has successfully helped hundreds of heart patients *reverse* their disease, and this without surgery. How? By putting them on a *self-help* program structured primarily around strict dietary changes, exercise, and stress-management techniques. He's empowering people to take charge, get well, and stay well. In so doing, he's become a leading spokesman for both the prevention and reversal of diet-and-lifestyle–related disease.

YOUR BODY, YOUR RESPONSIBILITY

There are, indeed, a growing number of professionals in a wide spectrum of health-care specialties who can teach and assist you in your health quest. In the end, however, the application of nutrition and other healthy habits is your responsibility alone. No one else *can* do the job for you. No one else *should* do the job for you. Your body is a gift from your Creator. It's yours to value and care for.

"Good health does not come easily; you must work for it," observes Dr. Charles B. Simone, author of *Cancer and Nutrition*.[14] Unfortunately, many of us don't start working on our health until we're faced with a major crisis. For some, that is too late. For instance, "half the people suffering a heart attack never reach the hospital alive."[15] It's much easier to prevent a killer disease before it happens than to try to regain your health once it's taken its toll. Death is a condition notoriously hard to reverse.

Don't neglect your responsibility to cultivate good health. Like it our not, you and I are going to have only one body in this life. Like the popcorn you buy at the movies, you'll want it to last through the whole show. Since most of us have many things on our script we hope to accomplish before the credits are run, these bodies of ours are going to have to last us a good long time. It is vitally important that we don't take our health for granted. If we do, we may be observing life from backstage—or bowing out early.

2
PLAN
"FEAST MEALS"

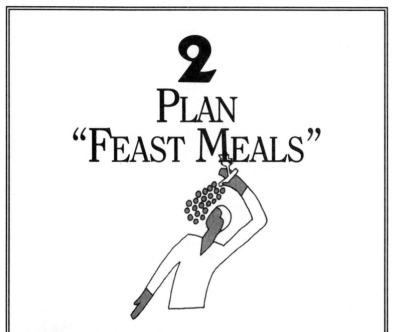

"Food, glorious food. . . ." So sang the orphans in the movie *Oliver*, based upon the novel about a young boy named Oliver Twist. They were held captive against their will in an orphanage by wicked masters who barely fed them, and getting more food was paramount in their thinking.

Indeed, eating is one of life's great pleasures. To be robbed of it strikes a severe blow to a person's psyche, as well as to his or her frame. Ever since man's stay in the original garden, food has been the centerpiece of celebrating our human existence. In the United States, food is the focal point for many of our social activities. Families get together around special meals, like Thanksgiving. Churches gather around potluck dinners and early-morning prayer breakfasts. Business people "do lunch" with each other as a way of taking care of more business.

Food is so key to our culture that even our individual identity is built around the kinds of food we prefer to consume. For instance, we talk about being "as American as the flag, baseball, and apple pie." We identify whole generations of people by the soda pop they drink. And we label ourselves or others as real "meat and potatoes" type people.

Given the reality that the kinds of foods we choose to eat is a central theme in our daily lives, any suggestion of change is met with significant resistance. With more than a little antagonism in his voice, a friend recently announced to me, "I'd rather die early, a happy man, than give up the foods I really enjoy." Of course, he'd never really seen anyone get eaten alive over a period of months or years by cancer. If he had, he'd have realized that one does not necessarily die happy. Nor had he stopped to consider how much more pleasant and satisfying his life could've been right then and there had his body and health been in better condition.

Perhaps like my friend, you too are more interested in enjoying the fullness of life right now than in living to a ripe old age. Quality over quantity. If that's true, then this book is for you. For my goal is not to put more years in your life, but more life in your years. I want to help you experience the best health your body is capable of. The quality of your life depends upon it. If it just so happens that by applying the principles in this book you do happen to live a long and active life (and that's a pretty good bet), then that's icing on the carrot cake.

Don't let anybody fool you, your health is your most important possession. No matter what else you own, consume, or experience, your health is the most important determinant of the quality of your existence. With it, the world is yours. You can go where you want to go and accomplish the things you want to accomplish. Without it, life becomes a struggle—a constant battle to keep your head above water. And just as the quality of our life is built upon the foundation of good health, the quality of our health is built upon the kinds of foods we feed our bodies.

Food was meant to be enjoyed, and eating to be a pleasure. But the content of the standard American diet (SAD) is destroying our health. Besides the life-threatening cancers, circulatory diseases (heart attack, stroke, high blood pressure, etc.), and diabetes that are closely tied to our typical diet, our society is ravaged by the less threatening but painful problems of headaches, allergies, skin problems, arthritis, yeast infections, respiratory problems, osteoporosis and bone fractures, obesity, hypoglycemia, and tooth decay. These maladies are among a host that are closely linked to the kinds of foods we feed ourselves.

A new diet needs to characterize our culture, one in which fat, sugar, and highly processed products are not the key ingredients. Even more important than a cultural change, however, is our individualized diet and lifestyle "retooling." Believe it or not, life doesn't lose its pleasure just because you scratch certain foods from your regular menu. Anne and I, along with countless others, have discovered a whole new world of taste sensations, and in the process have discovered that feeling healthy and clean inside has emotional and psychological benefits that can't be measured.

At the same time, acknowledging the reality that the changes presented in this book may be difficult at first to make, let me suggest that the very first thing you consider doing is to establish one meal a week where you can eat anything you desire. A once-a-week "feast meal" can be an important ally to the change process.

MOTIVATION

The principle behind this weekly indulgence involves motivation. If you begin to feel deprived of certain foods, you will quite likely lose the emotional motivation you need to keep going toward long-term health-promoting changes. There is a huge psychological difference between telling yourself you can *never* again eat such and such, as opposed to giving yourself freedom within certain boundaries. Besides, those who study nutrition tell us that it's not what we eat 5 percent of the time that'll kill us, but the stuff we feed our bodies the other 95 percent of the time.

One meal a week, out of twenty-one—that's just about right. That is, of course, if you're not in the throes of a special diet designed specifically to combat a particular disease. If so, it's important that you not deviate from the guidelines of your specific nutritional plan until your battle is won. But for those of us not in such a position, the one meal "off" a week can help to combat motivation-squelching feelings of deprivation.

In our own home we've been practicing the "feast meal" concept for several years now. Looking back, we note two distinct stages.

Stage one: Setting aside one meal at which we could eat "whatever" did help motivate each of us to stick to health-promoting foods for the rest of the week. At the same time, the postponement of cravings also seemed to actually intensify them at first. The pleasures of all those foods we made taboo in our daily regimen became exaggerated in our minds. Our Friday night "feast meals" were passionately anticipated. Like the kids in the poem who anxiously awaited Christmas morning, visions did dance in our heads. But instead of sugarplums, ours took the form of pizzas, chips, French fries, chocolate bars, pastries, pies, and ice cream.

When Friday nights finally rolled around, and none too soon, we'd load a shopping cart with these fantasy foods, throw in a couple of videos, and head home for a night of magnificent indulgence. Of course, Friday night sleep was always miserable, not to mention the headaches, gas pains, skin eruptions, weight gain, foul breath, constipation, and general crabbiness on Saturday. So much for magnificence. Slowly but surely, the pleasures attached to those foods we craved most began to wane.

Stage two: As we continued to see the various healthy eating habits described in this book take root in our lives, combined with the misery we'd feel on Saturdays, the compulsion to "junk out" on Friday nights steadily diminished. Our tastes changed, our attitudes adjusted. All of us, including our two kids, Jessica and Ben (fourteen and eleven, respectively, at the time of this writing), gave up meat and dairy products, except butter and an occasional cheese pizza on Friday nights. Our health improved dramatically. Our kids' bimonthly visits to the doctor for antibiotics against strep throat came to a halt. My headaches took a hike. Anne's immune system kept on getting stronger and stronger—this even in the aftermath of a vigorous battle with so-called terminal cancer that trashed her immune system and nearly cashed in her chips.

Yes, we do continue to feast once a week, but without the sense of passionate craving, and often (but not always) incorporating foods that would be considered nutritionally okay. This idea of a "feast meal" once a week is not set in cement. It's been working for us, but you need to tailor a plan that will work for you. The goal is to design a strategy that will keep you motivated to move continually toward better eating and optimal health the rest of the week. After you've read this book and have begun to implement some of the changes it suggests, see if the "feasting" concept helps you stay with your changes. You may need to start with two or three feast meals a week in order to maintain enthusiasm. Then again you might be the sort who prefers complete withdrawal from the kinds of foods that are less than health-promoting in order to avoid periodic arousal of those cravings. Do what works best for you. If you find something that works better than this once-a-week feast meal, write and tell us about it.

KEY QUOTES

Our eating habits are so deeply ingrained that there's not much chance of our developing a new diet against our will. . . . To make any kind of diet work for you, you need to know what you will eat, what you won't, and what you feel deprived without.
Lisa Tracy
The Gradual Vegetarian

Neither Rome nor a healthy lifestyle can be built in a day. . . . Developing a healthy lifestyle requires consistency, not perfection.
Gordon S. Tessler, Ph.D.
Lazy Person's Guide to Better Nutrition

A person can succeed at anything for which there is enthusiasm.
Charles M. Schwab

3
DRINK PURE WATER

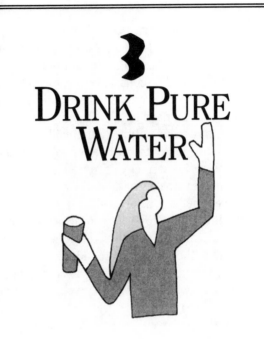

Water is a fundamental nutrient for human life. It is necessary to every system of our bodies. Not only does it play host to the millions of chemical reactions that happen in our bodies every second, but it serves to keep our joints moving, our nutrients flowing, our body temperature regulated, and acts as a solvent to remove waste products from the 70 trillion or so cells constantly at work within us. And you thought water was just for quenching thirst or washing down Aunt Trudy's chocolate cement cake!

Roughly 70 percent of our body weight is water. In an adult this boils down to about 12 gallons, requiring consumption of about 10,600 gallons over a lifetime to maintain.[1]

A rule of thumb for knowing how much you should consume each day is to divide your weight by two. This reflects the total number of ounces. Divide this by eight to get the number of glasses. It is a fact that the average American may well be chronically dehydrated and not even know it.

WHY DRINK PURE WATER?

We do need a steady supply of good old H_2O to keep our systems functioning at peak performance. However, when it comes to keeping our bodies well supplied, not just any water will do. In this section we will tell you why.

Pollution

In the United States today, much of our water comes from polluted sources. Here are just a few of the hundreds of examples that could be cited:

- 9.7 billion pounds of industrial chemicals are legally released into U.S. waters every year, according to Environmental Protection Agency (EPA) estimates.[2]
- In a recent EPA survey, nitrate (a carcinogen) showed up in more than half of the drinking-water wells tested across the country.[3]
- Seventy-four different kinds of pesticides have been found in drinking wells in thirty-eight states.[4]
- Four out of every five of the nation's one thousand worst hazardous waste dumps are leaking toxins into the ground water.[5]
- As many as 25 percent of the country's 2.5 million underground gasoline storage tanks, the kind found at every neighborhood gas station, are leaking gas into the local ground water, according to EPA estimates.[6]
- The 30 million acres of lawn in this country receive two and a half times more pesticides per acre than farm crops. These toxic chemicals find their way into local water supplies.[7]
- New York City dumps 1 million gallons of raw sewage a day into the Hudson River (an improvement from fifteen years ago when it was 450 million gallons a day).[8]

Chlorine

Ironically, in order to kill some of the live microorganisms in our water before we drink it, even more dangerous chemicals are added. Perhaps the most troublesome is chlorine.

First added to drinking water in the United States in the early 1900s, chlorine was used in an effort to control the spread of deadly diseases like typhoid and cholera. However, in the 1970s chlorine was identified as a potential health hazard. It was discovered that this potent chemical reacts with organic material in water, such as leaves and other decaying vegetation, to produce hundreds of chemical byproducts known as "trihalomethanes," or THMs. These are suspected of causing birth defects and certain kinds of cancer if consumed regularly in drinking water.

According to a recent article in *U.S. News and World Report*, "Drinking chlorinated water may as much as double the risk of bladder cancer, which strikes about 40,000 people a year."[9]

Fluoride

Dean Burk, chief chemist emeritus of the U.S. National Cancer Institute, states that "fluoride causes more human cancer death, and causes it faster, than any other chemical."[10]

Dr. Allen E. Banik, author of *The Choice Is Clear*, contends that "fluoridation not only hardens teeth, it also hardens the arteries and brain." He goes on to say that "Fluoridation of public drinking water is criminally intolerant, utterly unscientific, and chemical warfare."[11]

Nevertheless, the debate goes on. Should we continue to put fluoride in our drinking water or not? When it was first discovered in the early twentieth century that fluorides could help prevent tooth decay, adding it to our water supply seemed like a good idea. But do we really know what the accumulation of fluoride in our systems is doing to us?

In his book *Choose to Live*, Joseph D. Weissman, M.D., writes:

> The amounts of fluorides added to most water supply systems do not approach toxic levels. ... However, in addition to fluoride from drinking water, we get fluorides and fluorine compounds from other sources, at levels

that are usually not measured, with effects that are impossible to predict. Since fluorides exist throughout nature and have proliferated through industrial use in superphosphate fertilizers, plastics, refrigerants, toothpaste, and medicinal products, it is quite possible that people are exceeding safe levels of intake.[12]

Fluoride is a very potent poison that is suspect as a factor in bone diseases, including cancer.[13] New studies are also beginning to surface that seem to indicate that long-term, low-level consumption of fluoride in drinking water may be linked to increased susceptibility to hip fractures in older adults.

Lead
Not only is our water coming from polluted sources and then further contaminated by carcinogenic additives like chlorine and fluoride, but the delivery system through which it travels to our sinks and drinking fountains can add to the health hazards of ordinary tap water. As Dr. Weissman points out, "Water is a solvent, and as it travels through plastic, asbestos-lined concrete, or metal pipes containing soldered joints, it can absorb polyvinyl chloride, asbestos, lead, and cadmium, all of which are toxic. This is a problem even in those areas of the country that pride themselves on 'good' water."[14]

Of these toxic substances that can be leached from pipes, lead seems to be the one most often mentioned in literature dealing with plumbing concerns. In fact, the words *plumbing* and *lead* have something in common. Andrew Weil, M.D., points out that "our word plumbing comes from the Latin plumbum, meaning 'lead,' which is why the chemical symbol for this element is Pb."[15] He goes on to observe, "For most of history, water has flowed from reservoirs to kitchen taps through lead pipes, and even when copper or galvanized piping was used, connections were made with lead solder."

In 1986 the EPA did a study that discovered that more than 40 million Americans drink water that contains excessive levels of lead. That same year the further use of lead pipes and solder in plumbing was banned, although by then copper had become quite popular. If your home was built between 1910 and 1940, there is a good chance that you have lead pipes. This may also be true even of newer homes in the colder regions of the United States. For instance, lead plumbing was *required* in Chicago up until the 1986 ban.[16]

How much lead is excessive? Even minute quantities of lead in your water, as little as ten parts per billion, are enough to do harm to your body. Ideally, the level should not exceed five parts per billion. In kids and developing fetuses it can stunt growth, damage the nervous system, reduce intelligence, and cause severe retardation and death.[17] One in six kids under six years of age has elevated levels of lead in his or her blood, up to 40 percent of which comes from water.[18] Excessive lead in the blood of adults leads to high blood pressure and damaged organs.

Radon

According to *Consumer Reports* magazine, "Radon poses a greater health risk than any other environmental pollutant."[19] The EPA estimates that each year ten to forty thousand lung cancer deaths are attributable to breathing radon in our homes. It is a colorless, odorless, naturally occurring radioactive gas that forms as a byproduct of the breakdown of radium in the earth's crust. In most cases it enters and accumulates through cracks or holes in structural foundations. But it can also enter our homes via our tap water. Jospeh Cotruvo, director of the criteria and standards division of the EPA's Office of Drinking Water, contends that radon from tap water may be responsible for more deaths than all other drinking water contaminants combined.[20]

Water delivered directly from underground sources and not first exposed to the radon-dissipating effect of air is a threat, whereas water piped from lakes, rivers, and reservoirs is not. There are estimates that as many as 17 million people may have excessive levels of radon in their tap water.[21] If this is true at your house, it is released into your environment every time you get a drink, take a shower, wash dishes, or do laundry.

Parasites

Chlorine kills bacteria and viruses in our water supply, but not the parasites. The two most common, giardia and cryptosporidum, occur in water supplies as hard-shelled cysts that are chlorine-resistant. Thus, even if your source water is being disinfected, these "critters" are able to make it through to your tap. They can cause severe gastrointestinal problems in healthy people, while being life-threatening in people with impaired immune systems.[22]

KEY QUOTES

Tap water should be consumed internally only
for survival when good water is not available
and you are in danger of dehydration.
Joseph D. Weissman, M.D.
Choose to Live

The water we drink contains all manner of pesticides,
detergents, "optical brighteners," chemical salts,
fertilizers, human and animal excrement,
residues of heavy toxic metals,
dangerous chemicals and even radioactive wastes. . . .
Analysis of the water supplies of our large cities
have shown that not a single one of them
is free of every one of the chemicals known
to cause cancer in animals.
Harold W. Harper, M.D., and Michael L. Culbert
How You Can Beat the Killer Diseases

Tap water these days is more like soup, a chemical soup.
Harvey and Marilyn Diamond
Living Health

Unfortunately, water that may be hazardous to your health
may look, taste, and smell fine.
Health Letter Associates

HOW TO ENSURE PURE DRINKING WATER

What can you do on a practical basis to ensure that you're drinking the purest water possible? Some tips follow.

Get Your Water Checked

Start by asking your utility or public health department for a copy of its latest water analysis. However, that's only part of the story. More importantly, try to determine the quality of your water once it's made its way through the delivery system to your house.

Call upon the services of an independent, state-certified lab. Check your yellow pages under "Laboratories—Testing." Never ask a company that sells water-purifying equipment to test your water for you. The folks at *Consumer Reports* magazine liken that to asking a barber if you need a haircut. If you're unable to locate a lab near you, *Consumer Reports* (January 1990) recommends the following mail-order labs:

National Testing Laboratories
6151 Wilson Mills Road
Cleveland, OH 44143
(800)458-3330

WaterTest
33 S. Commercial Street
Manchester, NH 03101
(800)426-8378

Rudimentary Precautions

Here are three no-cost ways to reduce chlorine in your water:[23]

1. Let water stand in open, wide-mouthed containers for several hours. The chlorine will slowly be vaporized into the air.
2. Stir water in an uncovered blender or mixer for several minutes.
3. Boiling your water will help to remove residual chlorine, plus kill any microorganisms that might be in it.

Here are two no-cost ways to reduce the possibility of lead and other plumbing contaminants from your tap water.[24]

1. Let water run from the tap for a minute or two in the morning or after periods of nonuse. This flushes water that has had extensive contact with plumbing.

2. Never draw water from the hot-water tap for drinking or cooking. Hot water leaches out impurities much more readily than cold, and it's been sitting in a less-than-sterile hot-water tank. Dr. Weil contends that *"water from the hot tap is unfit for human consumption, no matter what your pipes are made of."*

Intermediate Provision
Purchase bottled water or water from a vending machine. Colin Ingram points out that there are basically five kinds of bottled water: *purified* or *distilled* water (contaminants and minerals removed); drinking water (contaminants removed, minerals left or replaced); fluoridated water (same as drinking water, fluoride added); *natural-source* water (not always safe, may contain toxic chemicals and metals); and *specialty* water (flavored natural-source or regular tap water).[25] (Note: There is significant debate as to whether or not water-borne minerals are necessary for human health. See below.)

1. If you plan to buy bottled water on a regular basis, go to the library and get a copy of the most recent *Consumer Reports* magazine that deals with this subject (January 1987, at the time of this writing). Know all you can and what you want before you buy.
2. Consider signing up with a company that will deliver pure drinking water to your home or office, in large glass bottles. Water is a solvent and tends to leach molecules from the plastic jugs it's often sold in.[26]
3. Many grocery and health-food stores now have their own "in-house" pure-water vending machines for use by customers. Look for a sticker on it that indicates certification and regular servicing. Most let you choose between drinking water or purified (distilled) water.

Advanced Protection
Purchase a water purifier for your home. There are three popular types, each made by several different companies. Get one

that will do what you need done, based upon your water tests. Either that, or get the one you feel most confident in.

Carbon filters (granular and block): Carbon granules are the size of coarse sand. Carbon block is very fine carbon pressed into a solid. The bigger the carbon filter and the more carbon involved, the better. This is because there is a direct relationship between the length of time water is in contact with the carbon and the purity of the final product. Thus the very small faucet-mount filters and the pour-through filters are much inferior to the larger high-volume filters.

At the same time, granular filters as a whole are inferior to carbon block. However, carbon block filters can become clogged with microscopic debris and rendered prematurely ineffective unless used with a sediment prefilter. They can also become a breeding ground for bacteria, as pollutants build up within the carbon.

A high-quality carbon block filter used in conjunction with a sediment prefilter will effectively remove most foul tastes and odors, organic chemicals, chlorine, and radon from your water.

Reverse osmosis systems: The reverse osmosis (RO) is a three-filter system. It has a prefilter that eliminates sediment; a reverse osmosis membrane through which water molecules are forced, leaving behind the larger pollutant molecules (organic chemicals, toxic minerals, radioactive minerals, and most microorganisms); and finally an activated carbon filter that does its thing with radon, chlorine, additional organic chemicals, plus tastes and smells.

RO systems do work slowly, but perhaps the greatest drawback to this sort of filtering system is the amount of water that most models waste. For every gallon of purified water produced, three to ten gallons are drained away with the pollutants.

Distillers: A distiller basically heats water into steam, then collects and cools it back into liquid. In the process pollutants are left behind. Distillation effectively removes the widest variety of contaminants from water. However, distillers do require an energy source, work even more slowly than RO systems, and give off a great deal of heat.

Dr. Banik contends that distilled water is "the only water which is pure. ... God's water for the human race."[27] For what it's worth, Dr. Weil says, "I packed up my home distiller for good after all the steam it gave off caused the paint to peel from my kitchen ceiling."[28] He now uses a reverse osmosis system.

The following summary is gleaned from Colin Ingram's exhaustive work *The Drinking Water Book*.[29]

REMOVAL SUMMARY	CARBON FILTERS	RO SYSTEMS	DISTILLERS
Tastes/Odors	Yes	Yes	Yes
Organic Chemicals *fertilizers, pesticides, herbicides, paints, fuels, cleansing agents, human and animal waste, etc.*	Yes	Yes	Yes
Additives *chlorine, fluoride*	Just chlorine	Yes	Yes
Inorganic Minerals/ Metals *calcium, magnesium, iron, manganese, aluminum, arsenic, asbestos, barium, cadmium, chromium, copper, fluoride, lead, mercury, nitrate, nitrite, selenium, silver*	No	Yes	Yes
Radioactive Substances *manmade radioactive minerals, radon gas*	Just radon	Yes	Yes
Microorganisms *bacteria, viruses, parasites*	No (yes in theory, no in practice)	Partial (all of them in theory, most of them in practice)	Yes

(Note: For information about specific brands and costs of each of these kinds of purifying systems, see the January 1990 edition of *Consumer Reports* magazine.)

KEY QUESTION

Q. I've heard that drinking distilled water tends to leach minerals from our bodies. If this is so, won't this cause a mineral deficit?

A. Dr. Allen E. Banik: "When it (rainwater) reaches the ground it is divinely designed to do one thing, to pick up minerals. These inorganic minerals are wonderful, but only for *plants*. The only minerals the body can utilize are the organic."[30] (In other words, our bodies can't utilize the inorganic minerals in water anyhow, so removing them from what we drink is no loss to our health.)

Harvey Diamond: "The body can use only organic minerals. . . . Anyone who knows biochemistry and physiology knows this to be true. . . . Your body can no more use an inorganic mineral than your car can run on Coca-Cola."[31]

Dr. Andrew Weil: "Water is not the source of your minerals. You get them from eating food, especially by eating a variety of vegetables. There is no truth to the belief that distilled water leaches minerals out of the body. The body is not like a metal pipe; it has elaborate ways to absorb, transport, and hold on to the various minerals it needs."[32]

Water is a vital nutrient for our bodies. For it to be health-promoting it must be pure. Avoid tap water. Buy bottled water or vending-machine water, or purchase a purifier for your home.

FURTHER READING

The Choice Is Clear by Dr. Allen E. Banik (Acres USA, P.O. Box 9547, Rayton, MO 64133). This forty-page booklet outlines the hazards of modern-day drinking water and the benefits of distilled water.

Choose to Live by Joseph D. Weissman, M.D. (New York: Penguin Books, 1988). See chapter 4: "Water and Beverages."

Clearer, Cleaner, Safer, Greener by Gary Null (New York: Villard Books, 1990). See chapter 4: "Water."

Consumer Reports magazine (January 1987). Reviews tests of fifty brands of bottled water.

Consumer Reports magazine (January 1990). Reviews home water purifiers and gives ratings of specific brands.

The Drinking Water Book by Colin Ingram (Berkeley, CA: Ten Speed Press, 1991). An excellent resource on different types of water-purifying systems.

Everyday Cancer Risks and How to Avoid Them by Mary Kerney Levenstein (Garden City Park, NY: Avery Publishing Co., 1992). See chapter 25: "Water."

Living Health by Harvey and Marilyn Diamond (New York: Warner Books, 1987). See chapter 7: "Water."

Living Well by Dale and Kathy Martin (Brentwood, TN: Wolgemuth and Hyatt, 1988). See chapter 7: "Cool, Clear, and Restful."

Natural Health, Natural Medicine by Andrew Weil, M.D. (Boston: Houghton Mifflin, 1990). See chapter 3: "What Will You Have to Drink?"

U.S. News and World Report magazine (29 July 1991). The cover page asks, "Is Your Water Safe?"

4
CUT DOWN ON FATS AND OILS

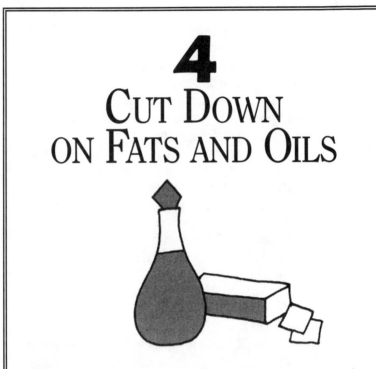

Ah, America, life in the "fats lane"! Statistics show that the average adult in this country may be consuming as much as 50 percent of his or her daily calories in food laden with health-destroying fats.[1]

Meat and dairy products, big hitters in the standard American diet, are big on fat. They will be discussed in the next two chapters.

The surprise is that from the early 1900s till now, the lion's share of dietary-fat increases in the typical American diet has come from fats and oils—things like vegetable shortening, margarine, and refined salad and cooking oils.[2]

Fats and oils are often categorized together under the single term *fats*. As you read the rest of this chapter, please keep that in mind. The world of fats can be a confusing one, and yet your health depends upon a good, basic understanding.

Let me see if I can't melt down a ton of information into a few basic facts to help you keep your fats (and oils) straight.

FAT FACTS

Fats are found in both the animal and plant kingdoms. In fact, every living thing contains some amount of fat. This is true because all cell membranes (both animal and plant) contain fatty acids.[3]

Fats are mixtures of different fatty acids: saturated, monounsaturated, and polyunsaturated. They differ in their composition, depending upon which fatty acid predominates. For instance:

▶ Beef fat, classified as saturated = 7.1 grams per tablespoon also contains 6.0 grams monounsaturated plus 0.5 grams polyunsaturated.[4]

▶ Olive oil, classified as monounsaturated = 9.8 grams per tablespoon also contains 1.9 grams saturated plus 1.2 grams polyunsaturated.[5]

Saturated Fats

Saturated fat is the "bad boy" of the fat world, for the following reasons:

Excess cholesterol—Saturated fat stimulates your liver to overproduce cholesterol. Our bodies need cholesterol as building blocks for cell membranes, digestive juices, and sex hormones, but like many things, too much of a good thing is not good. One thing leads to another, and all of a sudden you've got a major health crisis on your hands.

Circulatory diseases—As all this cholesterol finds a home in our arteries, it begins to shut off the flow of blood and oxygen to our various organs and body parts. As a result, they begin to deteriorate. Nasty things happen, depending upon which arteries are being clogged, like chest pains, heart attacks, strokes, lung problems, gangrene in the legs, blindness, loss of hearing, sexual impotence.

Cancer—Diets high in saturated fats have also been linked to a number of cancers, including those of the colon and breast—the second and third most prevalent killers among cancers after lung cancer. Other types we could be developing as we eat our way through 140 to 170 grams of fat a day (the average daily consumption of an adult American)[6] include cancers of the gallbladder, pancreas, prostate, uterus, and ovaries—just to name a few.

Saturated fat, solid at room temperature, is predominant in animal fats such as butter and lard. Coconut and palm oils are also very high in saturated fat. And believe it or not, all margarines and vegetable shortenings, even though they are made from healthier oils, are saturated fat as finished products. They become so as a result of the hydrogenation process they undergo to become solids.

"In the process of making liquid corn oil, safflower oil, and all other 'polyunsaturated' oils into margarine," writes David Reuben, M.D., "they are transformed into plain, ordinary 'saturated' oils. That has to be one of the greatest unexposed scandals in history. By hardening the vegetable oils, the margarine sellers are offering you the very saturated fats they claim to be helping you avoid."[7]

And as long as we're talking about margarines and shortenings, you must be warned about another negative. When you heat a polyunsaturated vegetable oil you begin to change the nature of its fatty acids. High heat, which is used to make margarine and shortenings, forms substances in these products called "*trans*-fatty" acids. These unnatural substances, which our bodies cannot effectively use, have been linked to circulatory diseases and cancer.[8] Margarine and shortenings just don't have anything going for them nutritionally—in fact, they are damaging to our bodies. Unfortunately, many of the bakery products at our local supermarkets contain one or more of these products.

Polyunsaturated Fats
Polyunsaturated fats are better. These include oils like safflower, sunflower, corn, and soy. They have a couple of things going for them.

Low in saturated fat—Polyunsaturated fats are low in saturated fatty acids. Of these, safflower oil is lowest, with sunflower oil a close second.

High EFAs—Polyunsaturates as a group contain the most "essential fatty acids" (EFA) of any of the fats. EFAs are fats our bodies must have in order to maintain health, but cannot make, so they must get them from outside sources. There are two: linoleic acid (LA), otherwise known as Omega-6 fatty acid; and linolenic acid (LNA), referred to as Omega-3 fatty acid. Most polyunsaturates contain only the Omega-6. By the way, saturated fats contain no EFAs.

The "superunsaturates," which are part of the polyunsaturate family, contain the very most EFAs. These are oils that are used strictly as dietary supplements. The star among them is flax oil, home to good supplies of both Omega-3 and Omega-6 fatty acids.

Drawback—The major concern with the polyunsaturated fats is that the more unsaturated an oil is, the more sensitive it is to the effects of light, heat, and oxygen. One needs to be very careful in their use and storage. They should not be used in cooking. In fact, once opened and exposed to oxygen or light, they begin a process that will eventually turn them rancid if not used up within a few weeks. Rancid (spoiled) oils can set off a chemical reaction in the body that is severely damaging to otherwise healthy tissue.

Andrew Weil, M.D., observes, "The products resulting from these oxidation reactions are highly reactive molecules that can damage DNA and other vital components of cells. Diets high in polyunsaturated fats increase the risk of cancer, speed up aging and degeneration of tissues, and may aggravate inflammatory diseases and immune-system disorders."[9]

Another unfortunate reality about these fats is that they are usually sold in transparent containers. "Light is the greatest enemy of the essential fatty acids," writes Udo Erasmus, Ph.D., author of the highly regarded book *Fats and Oils*. "Light is worse than oxygen. It destroys oil 1000 times faster. . . . Any oil sold in a clear glass bottle is subject to light deterioration, and contains health-destroying" components.[10] Unless, of course, they were highly refined before being bottled. If so, they shouldn't be used for anything, anyhow. The more refined an oil, the more useless and damaging to the body.

"Oil should be fresh, unrefined (extra virgin), mechanically pressed (no chemical leaching involved), organically grown, and stored in dark containers," continues Dr. Erasmus. "Only the health food stores carry acceptable oils, and not all oils in health food stores are acceptable."

(Special note: After opening a bottle of oil, it is best to put a drop or two of vitamin E in it and keep it refrigerated. This will keep the oil fresh for long periods of time.)

Monounsaturated Fats

All the literature seems to point toward the monounsaturates as good, all-purpose oils to use in your kitchen. These are the olive and canola oils.

Canola oil, in particular, is the newest star in the world of fats. It is made from the rapeseed plant from the mustard family, and is the traditional cooking oil of China, Japan, and India. Canadian scientists are responsible for breeding a form of rapeseed plant in their own country. The name "canola" comes from the words "Canadian oil."

Both canola and olive oil are less susceptible to the negative effects of light, heat, and oxygen than are the polyunsaturates. Canola oil can be used in cooking with temperatures up to 375 degrees Fahrenheit (baking, stir-frying in a wok), while olive oil is stable up to 320 degrees Fahrenheit. It also adds flavor to salads and other cold foods.

Besides being the oil that has the least saturated fat, canola oil is a source for both Omega-6 and Omega-3 essential fatty acids. "If you use any oil, canola oil should be your choice."[11] So writes Dean Ornish, M.D., author of the best-selling book *Dr. Dean Ornish's Program for Reversing Heart Disease*.

KEY QUOTES

When I was discussing fats with a group of medical students and mentioned solid vegetable shortenings, one student asked, "Why do they call it shortening?

What does it shorten?" Before I could respond,
another student answered, "Your life."
Andrew Weil, M.D.
Natural Health, Natural Medicine

Diseases of fatty degeneration today kill upward of 75%
of the people living in the affluent,
industrialized nations of planet Earth before their natural
"three score years and ten" are up. . . . It doesn't take
a genius to realize that if we want to get to the root
of the problem of fatty degeneration, we ought
to look at the whole field of fats and oils.
Udo Erasmus, Ph.D.
Fats and Oils

With all the importance Americans place on protein, it may
surprise you to learn that, as a percentage of daily calories,
we eat three to four times more fat than protein.
Jane Brody
Jane Brody's Nutrition Book

Of all the macronutrients in a rich diet, excess fat causes
the greatest burden on the body. Eventually the body fails
to compensate for this burden and disease results.
John A. McDougall, M.D.
The McDougall Plan

HOW TO CUT BACK

1. *First, rid your diet of as much saturated fat as possible.* If you consume butter or margarine on a regular basis, replace both with an intermediate product called "better butter." Blend together two sticks of butter with one cup of canola oil. Keep it refrigerated.

2. *Develop the habit of reading labels.* Be on your guard for hidden fats in processed foods. Health professionals are warning us to eliminate saturated fats and to reduce our over-

all intake of fat from 50 percent to 20 percent of our daily calo-ries.[12] If you're one who consumes the national average of 2,500 calories or so a day, this means no more than 500 of those should be in the form of fats—that's approximately 55 grams, or four tablespoons.

3. *Make the switch from a frying pan to an electric wok.* These use less heat and less oil. Put a little water in first, then the vegetables, then the oil.

FURTHER READING

Dr. Dean Ornish's Program for Reversing Heart Disease by Dean Ornish, M.D. (New York: Ballantine Books, 1990). See "Fat, Protein, Carbohydrate, and Cholesterol," pages 255-270.

Fats and Oils by Udo Erasmus (Vancouver, Canada: Alive Books, 1986).

Natural Health, Natural Medicine by Andrew Weil, M.D. (Boston: Houghton Mifflin, 1990). See "Fats," pages 16-25.

The Power of Your Plate by Neal D. Barnard, M.D. (Summertown, TN: Book Publishing Co., 1990). See "Fats and Oils," pages 56-59.

5
CUT DOWN ON MEAT OF ALL KINDS

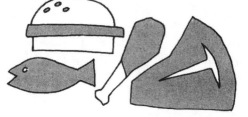

"Beef, real food for real people?" James Garner, a well-known Hollywood actor, had been hired by the advertising committee of the beef industry to deliver a similar message (one without the question mark) to the living rooms and kitchens of our homes. Ironically, as the ads were filling our television screens, Garner found himself filling a hospital bed, destined for coronary bypass surgery. Fortunately he recovered. In the light of his bout with serious heart disease, however, he changed his diet and opted to do car commercials rather than push beef.

As Neal D. Barnard, M.D., so cleverly puts it in his book *The Power of Your Plate*, "The moral of this story is if you're a 'real person' eating that kind of 'real food' you should live real close to a real good hospital, because you are likely to have very real problems."[1]

WHY CUT DOWN?

And it's not just red meat that's the problem, either. The health professionals are warning us that if we want to live long and healthy lives, we should cut back on meat of all kinds. What follows are some reasons.

Cholesterol
Cholesterol is a waxy substance that is important to the health and well-being of our bodies. It's a necessary building block in cell membranes, digestive juices, and sex hormones. However, we produce quite enough of it without adding more from an outside source.

All animal products contain cholesterol. The typical American diet, with meat at its core, burdens our bodies with unwanted and unusable cholesterol. Unless our bodies can somehow get rid of it, cholesterol deposits itself in our arteries. As it builds up, all kinds of nasty things can happen, depending upon which organs are being affected—things like heart attacks, strokes, gangrene in the legs, sexual impotence, loss of hearing and eyesight, and more.

I did say that all meat contains cholesterol. This includes such supposed dietary "do-gooders" as poultry and fish. To their credit, these meats are lower in saturated fat than red meats. However, based upon the number of calories consumed, they actually contain more cholesterol. To illustrate this fact, the following chart is adapted from Dr. John A. McDougall's book *McDougall's Medicine: A Challenging Second Opinion.*[2]

FOOD	MILLIGRAMS OF CHOLESTEROL PER 100 CALORIES
Lamb	21
Pork	24
Beef	29
Turkey (skinned)	43
Chicken (skinned)	44
Halibut	50
Mackerel	50
Tuna	50
Haddock	76
Crab	108
Shrimp	165
Liver	214
Lobster	278

According to Dr. McDougall, the higher cholesterol content of poultry and fish actually serves to negate the positive effects they might have as reduced saturated fat substitutes for red meat.

Saturated Fat

If cholesterol is accompanied by high levels of saturated fat, look out! You've got double trouble!! Besides the cholesterol in the meat, the saturated fat it contains stimulates your liver to produce its own cholesterol, creating a real "traffic jam" in your arteries.

It can begin early in life. John McDougall, M.D., notes, "Every child who has been raised on the high fat, high cholesterol American diet, which offers plentiful amounts of cow's milk, cheese, hot dogs, hamburgers, milk shakes, and french fries has signs of this disease by the tender age of 3."[3]

Typical Americans eating the standard American diet will have considerable build-up in their arteries before they're old enough to vote. Examinations of young American soldiers killed during the Korean and Vietnam wars showed "significant atherosclerosis (hardening of the arteries due to cholesterol build up) at only 18-20 years of age. Their Asian counterparts had much healthier arteries . . . the Americans had been eating lots of meat and dairy products all their lives, while the Asians had been eating mainly rice and vegetables."[4]

Beef, mutton, and pork all have the "double whammy" of cholesterol accompanied by high levels of saturated fat. (Poultry and fish, as was already noted, have less saturated fat but more cholesterol.)

Some kinds of fish do contain significant levels of two highly unsaturated fats that have been known to help protect arteries. These fats are called EPA and DHA and are part of the Omega-3 family of essential fatty acids. The molecules in these fats have such a strong tendency to want to move away from each other that they help to disperse cholesterol and other fatty-acid build-up in arteries. These fats have also shown themselves valuable in the treatment of cancer and arthritis. Johanna Budwig, M.D., has become world renowned in nutrition circles for her use of rainbow trout in successfully dissolving tumors in cancer patients.

Not all fish contain EPA and DHA. The best sources are salmon, sardines, mackerel, trout, tuna, eel—and to a lesser extent pike, carp, and haddock.[5] But before you run out and stock up on fish, finish reading this chapter. There are other things to take into consideration.

High Protein

Everybody is different. Every one of us comes equipped with an individualized biological blueprint. It's quite impossible to predict for certain exactly what a high-protein diet will eventually do to your particular health picture. But by reducing your consumption of all types of meat now, you can reduce your potential risk of developing some very nasty degenerative diseases that have been associated with high-protein diets.

Cancer—We all have cancer cells floating around in us from time to time. They are malfunctioning or otherwise mutant cells, a part of the biology of life and nothing to worry about, unless of course our immune system, which destroys them, is not functioning properly. A high-protein diet built around meat has the potential to weaken our immune systems. According to nutritionist Maureen Salaman, the pancreatic enzymes which we need to digest meat also play a role in our immune forces to help protect us from the build-up of cancer cells. These enzymes actually attack the protein coating that surrounds a cancer cell. The more meat we eat, the fewer pancreatic enzymes we have available to go after cancer cells.[6]

In his book *Healing Nutrients*, Patrick Quillin, Ph.D., cites a large study done in Germany that found a link between high protein intake and the risk of developing cancer of the pancreas itself. He goes on to note that the "average American consumes about 50 percent more protein than recommended levels." Not only is pancreatic cancer a concern, but so is cancer of the colon. "High-meat diets are known to elevate the risk for colon cancer," observes Quillin, "possibly due to the intestinal bacteria that thrive on meat and create DNA-altering materials as a result."[7]

I'm not trying to scare you; I'm just presenting the facts you need to know as you consider how to take the best care of the body you've been given.

Osteoporosis—The high protein found in meat-based diets can contribute to the development of osteoporosis, a condition in which teeth become soft and bones become dangerously weak and brittle because of loss of calcium. Medical science now realizes that the more protein we eat, the more calcium we lose.

Dr. McDougall writes, "I would like to emphasize that the calcium-losing effect of protein on the human body is not an area of controversy in scientific circles. The many studies performed during the past 55 years consistently show that the most important dietary change we can make if we want to create a positive calcium balance that will keep our bones solid is to decrease the amounts of protein we eat each day."[8]

Kidney failure—Because high-protein diets cause calcium to be released from our bones, this calcium eventually finds its way via our bloodstreams to our kidneys. Here it can form stones, destroy tissue, and otherwise impair function.

In addition to dealing with all this released calcium, your body must also deal with the excess protein consumed in a meat-centered diet. What it can't put to use immediately, it must get rid of. Studies show that the average American consumes more than five times the amount of protein he or she needs each day.[9] (More about this at the end of this chapter.) Excessive protein puts significant stress on our kidneys. People who have eaten meat all their lives tend to have kidney problems in their later years.

"Forcing your kidneys to filter and excrete 50 to 100 grams of unnecessary protein daily is like driving your car at 8,000 RPM when it was designed to be driven at 3,500," observes Julian M. Whitaker, M.D.[10]

Acid Production
All foods are either acid or alkaline forming in our bodies. Our systems are always at work, trying to keep the proper acid/alka-

line balance in our blood. If our diets contain a lot of meat, which by its nature is acid forming, our bodies are forced to draw calcium (an alkaline mineral) from our bones to help restore the slightly alkaline pH level our blood requires. Thus the acid-forming nature of meat in our digestive system, along with the calcium-robbing effect of its protein, provides a one-two punch to our bones and teeth.

Production Chemicals and Drugs
Current practices in livestock and poultry management are producing meat products that are laden with production chemicals and drugs that undermine human health. These substances, unlike bacteria, which can be killed by cooking, remain in the animal products when consumed by humans.

Antibiotics—Half of the more than 31 million pounds of antibiotics produced each year in the United States are mixed into the feeds of cows, pigs, and chickens.[11] They are used to improve growth rates and to fight off infections that run rampant in factory-type farming where animals are crowded together in confined quarters. The question is, what do these drugs do to you, the consumer, when steadily ingested through a meat-centered diet?

> ▶ Exposure to toxic substances—Sulfamethazine, a drug commonly used, is a suspected carcinogen in humans.[12]
> ▶ Allergic reaction—Residue drugs found in both meat and dairy products have the potential to cause serious reactions in people who are allergic to penicillin.[13]
> ▶ Antibiotic-resistant bacteria in our bodies—There is concern that the antibiotic residues stored up in the meat we eat will serve to develop strains of drug-resistant bacteria in our bodies over time. If any of these bacteria lead to an infection at some point, antibiotics would be rendered ineffective. Then what do you do?! "Only a few effective antibiotics are available for treating some very serious infections. If you happen to get

one of those infections, and it is caused by bacteria that are resistant to these antibiotics, the results could be fatal."[14]

Growth hormones—Livestock are also routinely pumped full of hormones to fatten them up quickly for market. One of these, the female hormone estrogen, is considered by many a likely contributor to the onset of cancer, ovarian cysts, and premature sexual development in children.[15]

Environmental Contaminants

Polluted conditions in the environment cause many of the meat products humans consume to contain concentrated amounts of disease-causing contaminants. In his book *Choose to Live*, Joseph D. Weissman, M.D., writes that "animal products are the single largest source of pesticides in the human diet." He goes on to point out that "we obtain from meat 16 times the amount of pesticides we would from an equivalent amount of plant food."[16]

Contamination is "*least* concentrated in root vegetables, grains, legumes, fruits, and leafy vegetables. It is *more* concentrated in oils and fats and dairy products. It is *most* concentrated in the flesh and fowl that eat these things, reaching its *ultimate* concentration in man, who feeds on fat animals and fish that already have concentrated chemical pollutants in their tissues."[17]

A Few Fish Stories

▶ A study done by the FDA in 1983 found that 334 of 386 types of domestic fish in the United States contained DDT in their meat (a pesticide and probable human carcinogen), although DDT had by then been banned from agricultural use for eleven years.[18]

▶ A study done in 1986 found that 65 percent of cod (an ocean fish), 50 percent of crappie, and 98 percent of freshwater trout had cancerous tumors, the effects of contaminated waters.[19]

▶ A study done in 1992 at fish markets in Chicago and New York found "PCBs in almost 43 percent of the salmon, half the whitefish, and a quarter of the swordfish."[20] (PCBs are carcinogenic chemicals that were used as coolants, lubricants, and insulating fluids before being banned in 1979.)

▶ As we have seen earlier in this chapter, some fish do contain valuable Omega-3 fatty acids. Because of the problems of pollution, however, Dean Ornish, M.D., author of the best-selling book *Dr. Dean Ornish's Program for Reversing Heart Disease*, recommends vegetarian sources.[21] These include fruits, green leafy vegetables, whole grains, beans, seaweed, and soybean products.[22]

Nitrites and Nitrates
These chemicals, often found on labels as sodium nitrite or sodium nitrate, are added to processed meats such as ham, bacon, hot dogs, bologna, salami, corned beef, sausage, etc., in an effort to prevent spoilage and preserve color. When these compounds mix with a certain kind of chemical called "amines" that are found naturally in the stomach, "nitrosamines" are formed. These are highly potent cancer-causing agents.

The list could go on and on. Bottom line, be very careful about the kinds of meat products you choose, and cut way back on the quantity you consume. Treat meat as a delicacy, something to be enjoyed at feasts or on special occasions. The Bible talks about killing the fatted calf for special celebrations. Trouble is, we Americans insist on killing one every day for breakfast, another for lunch, and yet another for dinner. Meat eating is a learned habit, not a physical necessity. You may well want to consider saying goodbye to meat altogether.

KEY QUOTES

*A high-animal-protein diet, especially an excess of meat,
is definitely detrimental to the health*

and may be a contributor to or a direct cause
of the development of many of our most common diseases,
as shown by recent massive research.
Paavo Airola, Ph.D.
The Airola Diet and Cookbook

Historically, the eating of meat in any society has been
directly proportionate to its wealth and degree
of civilization. The amount of cancer has also appeared
in approximately the same proportions.
Maureen Salaman
The Cancer Answer . . . Nutrition

Even if you made no other changes in your eating habits,
you'd be in a far more favorable position in terms of cancer
risk if you simply ate less meat.
Donald R. Germann, M.D.
The Anti-Cancer Diet

A health-supporting diet contains no animal products.
John A. McDougall, M.D., and Mary A. McDougall
The McDougall Plan

HOW TO CUT DOWN

Cutting down on meat can be difficult for the average American. Perhaps you will want to consider changing your meat-eating habits in phases. Here are some thoughts and ideas:

Phase One: Exploration
Buy a vegetarian cookbook and start trying out some meatless recipes. If there are classes you can take on vegetarian cooking, do so. If you have friends who eat this way, exchange recipes and ideas. Also, sample the meat substitutes at your local health-food store.

You're building a whole new food culture. Changing cultures is always difficult, like moving to a new country. If at first you're frustrated, that's only par for the course. Keep going. Keep exploring. Go on to the next recipe, try the next product. As you find things you really like, keep track. Write them down. You're still eating meat, but you're also eating a few vegetarian meals.

By the way, make sure that whatever meat is still part of your diet at this point has been "organically" produced. In other words, the animals were raised free of many of the production chemicals and contaminants that have become commonplace in today's livestock production methods. Look for organic meat in health-food stores or see if it's available through your local grocer.

Phase Two: Substitution
You've already been eating some vegetarian meals. Now you want to begin to strategically substitute those you enjoy for the meat-based meals you need to cut back on. Design a one-week menu of meals incorporating some of your new vegetarian cuisine, leaving out red meat and processed meats.

At the same time, continue to explore additional vegetarian meal ideas. As you come across ones you enjoy, redesign your one-week master menu. Substitute these new meals for chicken and fish, or other meats you might be used to eating.

Phase Three: Integration
At this point you should have a fully developed one-week menu for vegetarian eating that you can live with. Don't stop there. Keep exploring meal possibilities. Keep exchanging recipes and ideas with others. Keep trying new things. Integrate all that you learn and discover into your new food culture. Enlarge your master menu to two weeks, and beyond. Variety is the spice that will keep your new way of eating alive and exciting.

KEY QUESTIONS

Perhaps no questions in the field of health and nutrition draw more debate than those surrounding the issue of protein. The RDA for protein in average men and women has been put at 56 grams and 44 grams, respectively. Fifty-six grams is only about two ounces a day. Many nutrition-minded physicians and scientists contend that even this is much more than our bodies really need, since on the average we tend to lose only about 23 grams (less than one ounce) each day. As was already pointed out concerning protein, more is not necessarily better. With this in mind, let's pick off some of the questions you undoubtedly have and see if we can't get at some simple answers.

Q. If I cut back on or eliminate meat, where will I get my protein?

A. First of all, you need to understand amino acids. Human beings build human protein by breaking down protein-containing foods into their amino acid components. In other words, you don't build protein by eating protein, but by how well your body is able to digest food and utilize amino acids.

Q. Okay, but do plants contain the kinds of amino acids I need?

A. Harvey Diamond: "There are 23 different amino acids . . . 15 can be produced by the body and 8 must be derived from the foods we eat. Only these 8 are called *essential*. If you eat any fruits, vegetables, nuts, seeds, or sprouts on a regular basis, you are receiving all the amino acids necessary for your body to build the protein it needs . . . and although all fruit and vegetables contain most of the 8, there are many fruits and vegetables that contain *all* the amino acids not produced by the body: carrots, bananas, brussels sprouts, cabbage, cauliflower, corn, cucumbers, eggplant, kale, okra, peas, potatoes, summer squash, sweet potatoes, and tomatoes. Also all nuts, sunflower and sesame seeds, peanuts, and beans contain all 8 as well."[23]

Q. But won't I have to eat an enormous amount of plant food in order to get enough amino acids to build the protein I need?

A. A lot less than you think. Let's say just for the sake of illustration that your need is 56 grams of protein each day.

That's equivalent to one cup broccoli (5 grams), ½ cup raw sunflower seeds (17 grams), two cups cooked brown rice (13 grams), one cup cooked lentils (16 grams), and one cup cooked oatmeal (5 grams). And as I said, many, like Doctors McDougall and Weissman below, contend that we need much less protein than that each day.

John A. McDougall, M.D.: "At most, an adult needs no more than 20 grams of protein a day, or about two-thirds of an ounce. . . . Most Americans consume 105 to 120 grams and more of proteins each day. . . . Starchy foods, most vegetables, and almost all fruits have protein contents that are the most sensible for humans to eat."[24]

Joseph D. Weissman, M.D.: "It is virtually impossible to develop a protein deficiency on a vegetarian diet. Vegetables, legumes, grains, nuts, and seeds contain more than enough protein for the body's growth and maintenance."[25]

Q. But I've heard that vegetable protein is not complete protein—that the pattern of amino acids these foods provide needs to be properly combined in order to be adequate. Do I need to be careful to eat these foods in a certain way to make them so?

A. First of all, we've already seen that there are a variety of fruits and vegetables which provide all eight essential amino acids in and of themselves from which human protein can be manufactured. That, in itself, should calm any fears that plant proteins are decidedly inferior to animal proteins.

Second, much of the strict emphasis some still hold concerning plant protein combining stems from a book written in the late 1960s by a woman named Frances Moore Lappe. It was entitled *Diet for a Small Planet* and was an attempt to show that we don't actually need animal protein in our diets in order to build healthy bodies. She spent a great deal of the book (200 out of 280 pages) outlining in detail how combining certain plant proteins together could make them equivalent to the protein content of an egg.

But was the egg the ideal protein food? Nathan Pritikin was one of many nutritionists who believed not, based upon his own clinical studies to the contrary. He considered the book misleading. "Unfortunately, the book is one of the most misleading documents in the last few years because everybody now thinks food balancing is essential. . . . [The book] gives the impression that vegetable proteins don't have sufficient percentages of amino acids."[26]

Not only that, but Lappe's readers came away with the impression that the process of combining plant protein just right took the brains of a rocket scientist and the precision of a brain surgeon.

Ten years and much study later, Lappe rewrote *Diet for a Small Planet*. Of the 455 pages in its new form, only about sixty dealt with the concept of plant protein combining, and much of this was an explanation of how her thinking had changed on the subject. In this tenth anniversary edition she included this remarkably humble statement:

> In 1971 I stressed protein complementarity because I assumed that the only way to get enough protein . . . was to create a protein as usable by the body as animal protein. In combating the myth that meat is the only way to get high-quality protein, I reinforced another myth. I gave the impression that in order to get enough protein without meat, considerable care was needed in choosing foods. Actually, it is much easier that I thought. . . . [I] helped create a new myth—that to get the protein you need without meat you have to conscientiously combine nonmeat sources. . . . With a healthy, varied diet, concern about protein complementarity is not necessary for most of us.[27]

Julian M. Whitaker, M.D.: "It was commonly believed in the past that great effort was needed to 'balance' the vegetable proteins to form 'complete' protein. Most scientists now realize that a diversified vegetable diet will supply more than adequate protein for all our needs."[28]

Frances Moore Lappe (in the new edition of *Diet for a Small Planet*): "If people are getting enough calories, they are virtually certain of getting enough protein."[29]

Q. If I don't eat meat and at the same time do hard physical labor or compete athletically, shouldn't I supplement my diet with some sort of protein powder?

A. **David Reuben, M.D.:** "Protein serves the function of replacing enzymes, rebuilding blood cells, producing antibodies, and replenishing mucus, among other things. None of those elements are damaged by doing physical work. . . . Any protein you eat—beyond that approximate necessary ounce or so—will not make you stronger or happier or more attractive. It will not develop the breasts of women, increase the sexual potency of men, or make little children get better grades in school. These, and all the other claims made for protein, are designed to fortify the bank accounts of hustlers who peddle high-protein concentrates."[30]

Patrick Quillin, Ph.D., R.D.: "Muscles are composed primarily of protein and water. Tough connective protein (collagen and elastin) provides a cellular 'glue' to keep them durable. Vitamin C helps to build this connective protein. Vitamin B_6 helps to metabolize all proteins. Since muscles are largely protein, a longstanding myth has been that 'the more protein you eat, the bigger your muscles will get.' Not true. Muscle size depends more upon athletic training and genetic endowment. Most athletes eat too much protein. Excess protein can stress the kidneys and liver, drain calcium from the bone stores, and even cause weight problems."[31]

FURTHER READING

Diet for a New America by John Robbins (Walpole, NH: Stillpoint, 1987). See particularly chapter 7: "The Rise and Fall of the Protein Empire."

Fit for Life by Harvey and Marilyn Diamond (New York: Warner Books, 1985). See chapter 9: "Protein."

Healing Nutrients by Patrick Quillin, Ph.D., R.D. (Chicago: Contemporary Books, 1987). Information on protein is scattered throughout the book.

Living Health by Harvey and Marilyn Diamond (New York: Warner Books, 1987). See "The Case Against Meat," pages 220-224.

The McDougall Plan by John A. McDougall and Mary A. McDougall (Piscataway, NJ: New Century Publishers, 1983). See chapter 4: "Red Meat, Poultry, and Fish Are Avoided on a Health-Supporting Diet."

6

CUT DOWN ON ALL DAIRY PRODUCTS

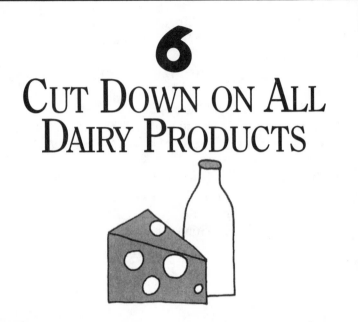

or nine years my wife and I made our home in beautiful Wisconsin—land of beer, bratwurst, and dairy products. They're crazy about their cheese up there, and it shows. Some of the fans at University of Wisconsin football games wear hats on their heads shaped like cheese wedges. Along one of the highways that dissects the state there's a statue of a giant mouse holding a big chunk of cheddar. I even met a native son one time who went by the name Cheese! Dairy farms dot the countryside. Making "moo juice" is big business. If there's any gold to be found in the state, it sits on the shelves in dairy cases.

Many of us have grown up, whether in Wisconsin or elsewhere, firmly believing that dairy products are some of the most nutritious foods we can eat. "Milk does a body good," our television sets tell us. It makes our muscles big, our teeth strong, and our bodies beautiful—at least according to the National Dairy Council.

And why should we doubt them? Milk is, after all, the perfect food. Isn't it?

WHY CUT DOWN?

If you'll step away from all the television commercials and all the hype and begin to look at what nutritionists and nutritionally aware physicians have been saying for years, you'll get a whole new picture about how dairy products impact our health. The truth is, we need to consider eliminating or cutting back on our consumption for the following reasons:

Lactose Intolerance

Much has been written about the fact that somewhere between birth and about four years of age, most people in this world lose the ability to digest cow's milk. There are two reasons for this: *lactase* and *rennin*. Lactase is the enzyme we need to break down the natural sugar in milk (lactose); rennin is the enzyme needed to break down the protein (casein).

"By age three or four rennin is nonexistent in the human digestive tract and, in all but a small number of people, so is lactase," explain Harvey and Marilyn Diamond in their book *Living Health*.[1] In other words, most of us (some say as many as 98 percent) simply don't have the digestive equipment to make productive use of cow's milk and most dairy products.

This, of course, leads to a wealth of health problems for a population, such as ours, that continues to hold the "udder truth" that what comes from dairy cows is a must in humans for strong bones and healthy bodies. So strongly do we believe that every year we collectively find our way through 75 billion pounds of dairy products—300 pounds per every man, woman, and child.[2] And we reap the consequences.

Allergic Reactions

The protein in dairy products has been implicated in a host of food allergies. In fact, cow's milk and the products made from it are the leading cause of food allergies in humans.

- ▶ *Gastrointestinal problems*—Canker sores, vomiting, colic, stomach cramps, abdominal distention, intestinal obstruction, bloody stools, colitis, malabsorption, loss of appetite, growth retardation, diarrhea, constipation, painful defecation, irritation of tongue, lips, and mouth.[3]

▶ *Respiratory problems*—The protein in milk causes increased mucus production in most people. This can be a significant contributor to the onset and severity of hay fever, asthma, bronchitis, sinusitis, colds, runny noses, and ear infections.[4]

▶ *Skin problems*—Rashes, atopic dermatitis, eczema, seborrhea, hives.[5]

▶ *Behavioral problems*—Irritability, restlessness, hyper-activity, headache, lethargy, fatigue, allergic-tension fatigue syndrome, muscle pain, mental depression, enuresis (bed wetting, often caused when the bladder tissues become swollen and insensitive to the feeling of fullness).[6]

▶ *Other potential allergic reactions*—Migraine headaches and iron deficiency anemia.

Saturated Fat and Cholesterol

Milk, like meat, supplies our bodies with things we don't need or want, namely saturated fat and cholesterol. In fact, milk is often referred to as "liquid meat," their macronutrient content being so similar.

What about using skim milk? The main problem is that when you take the fat out of any of the dairy products, the proteins and lactose become even more concentrated. As we have seen, these are the things in dairy products that cause so many of the health problems associated with them. It is for this reason that John A. McDougall, M.D., says that "skim milk and other low-fat dairy products are unacceptable in a health-supporting diet."[8]

Calcium-Robbing High Protein

Being high in protein, dairy products contribute to the onset of osteoporosis. As was explained in the chapter on meat, a high-protein diet robs our bodies of calcium. The typical American diet, high in meat and dairy, is a hotbed for osteoporosis—weak teeth and soft bones due to calcium loss.

The more milk you drink, even though it's high in calcium, the more calcium you will lose. John A. McDougall, M.D., points out, "Researchers estimate that doubling the amount of proteins in the diet will increase by 50% the amount of calcium lost in the urine."[9]

In other words drink *less* milk, not more, if you wish to have strong teeth and bones.

I know, I know. This flies in the face of all that you've been taught. But who taught you? Okay, your mother. But where did she learn what she thinks she knows about milk? Television— that's right. Or at school, where she was indoctrinated with the concept of the four food groups.

Guess who thought up that idea, sold the government on starting to promote it in all the schools back in the 1950s, and has been the leading producer of food "education" materials ever since? If you guessed The National Dairy Council, you'd be right.

One wonders why we rely on business, whose sole purpose it is to promote their products, to educate us on what is truly healthy. Did you ever stop to wonder why cheese showed up in two of the four basic food groups?

Acid Production

All foods are either acid or alkaline forming in our bodies. All dairy products, with the exception of butter, are acid producing. As was explained in the chapter on meat, our bodies are in a state of health when they are able to maintain a proper acid/alkaline balance in our blood.

The standard American diet (SAD), high in both meat (acid forming) and dairy (acid forming), puts a tremendous strain on our systems to balance these acidifying foods. Calcium is released from our bones and teeth to neutralize their effect. Is it any wonder that osteoporosis is a $4 billion dollar industry in the United States?[10] Fifteen to twenty million Americans are afflicted with this very avoidable disease, by no means a necessary part of growing old.

Other Potential Health Problems

▶ *Leukemia*—Twenty percent of dairy cows have leukemia viruses. In studies where other animals were fed cow's milk, it was shown that these become infected and develop leukemia. It could well be that these viruses are passed on to humans who drink cow's milk.[11]

▶ *Multiple Sclerosis*—Kids who are raised on cow's milk have been shown to develop a nervous system that is susceptible to disease later in life. In fact, MS is found most in parts of the world where infants and children are fed cow's milk as opposed to mother's milk and vegetable foods.[12]

▶ *Hodgkin's Disease*—Also known as cancer of the immune system, it can be caused by constant over-stimulation by dairy proteins.[13]

▶ *Colic*—A common allergic reaction in infants to dairy proteins passed on through mom's breast milk after she's eaten dairy products.[14]

▶ *Others*—Congestive heart failure in infants, prostate cancer, amyotrophic lateral sclerosis (Lou Gehrig's disease), rheumatoid arthritis, lupus, and insulin-dependent diabetes.[15]

Toxic Chemical Residues

By now you're probably wondering, why consume dairy products at all? If so, I've accomplished my objective. If you need more help being convinced to cut way back or give them up completely, there's always this to add:

Antibiotics—Dairy cows are routinely treated with antibiotics for infection of their udders. These drugs are passed on to humans through the cow's milk. Many people are dangerously allergic to antibiotics such as penicillin. Then, too, the more antibiotics we ingest with our food, the more resistant disease-producing bacteria in our bodies become to them. If we ever really need to use antibiotics orally at some point, their effectiveness will have been greatly hindered.

Pesticides—Detectable amounts of cancer-causing pesticide products have been found in pasteurized milk purchased in supermarkets. It only makes sense. The plants we feed our animals these days are sprayed with pesticides to fight off insects. These pesticides become concentrated in the fat of the animals, especially in the milk. Unlike bacteria, heat processing does not remove these chemicals. And so you and I eventually partake of what was originally meant to kill bugs.

KEY QUOTES

The dairy industry would like us to believe that we never outgrow our need for milk, and that milk is nature's most perfect food, but there are reasons to think otherwise.
Andrew Weil, M.D.
Natural Health, Natural Medicine

[Cow's] milk has no valid claim as the perfect food.
As nutrition, it produces allergies in infants,
diarrhea and cramps in the older child and adult,
and may be a factor in the development of heart attacks
and strokes. Perhaps when the public
is educated as to the hazards of milk,
only calves will be left to drink the real thing.
Only calves should drink the real thing.
Frank A. Oski, M.D.
Don't Drink Your Milk!

Dairy products are disease-producing.
They're harmful. They cause suffering.
They're the perfect thing to eat if you want to be sick
and have a diseased body.
Harvey and Marilyn Diamond
Living Health

In addition to the scientific and medical evidence against dairy products, we can observe the way milk is used

by other animals. No other animal in its natural
environment drinks milk after it is weaned.
Furthermore, in nature no young animal drinks
the milk of another species.
John A. McDougall, M.D., and Mary A. McDougall, L.P.N.
The McDougall Plan

Had enough? Here's one more quote that pretty much sums up why you should consider cutting way back on dairy products. It comes from Harvey and Marilyn Diamond, authors of *Fit for Life*, America's all-time number-one health and diet book:

Please do something about decreasing the amount of animal products you eat. The only reason you may *not* want to do so is that you are totally unconcerned about the possibility of developing cancer, leukemia, heart disease, heart attack, high blood pressure, high cholesterol levels, diabetes, arthritis, multiple sclerosis, thyroid impairment, goiter, ulcers, gout, kidney damage, liver damage, migraine headaches, gallstones, kidney stones, SIDS, tinnitus, asthma, allergies, ear infections, bronchitis, sinusitis, or osteoporosis.[16]

HOW TO CUT BACK

1. *Try milk substitutes.* Our family loves a product called Rice Dream, a milk made from rice. There are also several soy milk products on the market. Your supermarket may carry some of these, but your local health-food store is your best bet. Get them, try them out, pick one to stick with.

  2. *Try cheese substitutes.* There are many kinds of soy cheeses available at health-food stores. They're a bit of an acquired taste, as are all things in life.

  3. *Try better butter or butter substitutes.* Better butter is made by adding two sticks of butter with one cup of canola oil. By blending the butter with oil, you are in effect cutting down

on the amount of saturated fat you would get in a similar amount of just butter.

4. *Prepare banana ice cream.* Peel and freeze a handful of bananas. If you've got a juicer that can homogenize foods, put them through it. What you get is something that looks and tastes like soft-serve ice cream.

KEY QUESTION

Q. If I don't drink milk, where will I get my calcium?

A. John McDougall, M.D.: "Many green and yellow vegetables and fruits give plentiful amounts of calcium . . . all natural diets, including purely vegetarian diets without a hint of dairy products, contain amounts of calcium that are above the threshold for meeting your nutritional needs. In fact, the scientific literature states clearly that a 'calcium deficiency disease' due to a low calcium intake from natural diets simply does not exist."[17]

Joseph D. Weissman, M.D.: "Under ordinary circumstances, vegetable sources of calcium are adequate. Almost all diets contain calcium in amounts above the threshold of human needs; a diet lacking in calcium is virtually impossible to find."[18]

The amount of calcium needed in our diets on a daily basis has been a much-debated issue. The World Health Organization suggests 400 milligrams a day. In the United States, where we experience high rates of osteoporosis (weakening of the bones due to calcium loss), the recommended daily allowance (RDA) has recently been raised from 800 to 1,200 milligrams. Of course, if we just ate less protein, especially meat, the RDA would no doubt drop dramatically.

If you're eating any of the following on a regular basis, don't worry about a calcium deficiency, especially if you've cut back on meat: vegetables (especially broccoli), grains, beans, raw seeds (especially sesame seeds), nuts (especially almonds), and various kinds of seaweed (especially kelp).

In the end, "the most important dietary change that we can make if we want to create a positive calcium balance that will keep our bones solid is to DECREASE the amount of proteins we eat each day ... not to increase the amount of calcium we take in."[19]

FURTHER READING

The Book of Whole Foods: Nutrition and Cuisine by Karen MacNeil (New York: Vintage Books, 1981). See "Dairy Products," pages 211-248.

Don't Drink Your Milk by Frank A. Oski, M.D. (Syracuse, NY: Mollica Press, 1983).

Food and Healing by Annemarie Colbin (New York: Ballantine Books, 1986). Chapter 6, "The Effects of Different Foods," presents an excellent discussion concerning the health risks of dairy products, as well as some other foods typical to the American diet.

Living Health by Harvey and Marilyn Diamond (New York: Warner Books, 1987). See "The Case Against Dairy Products," pages 224-239.

The McDougall Plan by John A. McDougall, M.D., and Mary A. McDougall, L.P.N. (Piscataway, NJ: New Century Publishers, 1983). See "Dairy Products," pages 49-56.

Natural Health, Natural Medicine by Andrew Weil, M.D. (Boston: Houghton Mifflin, 1990).

7
EAT LOTS OF RAW, ORGANIC FRUITS AND VEGETABLES

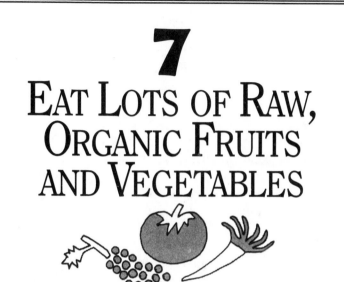

"Ode to the Produce Section"
by Dave Frähm

At my favorite store, daytime or night,
Laid out before me, a delectable sight.
Carrots and peppers and onions, galore,
Melons and peaches and oranges, and more.

A carpet of colors, a feast for the senses,
They build up your cells, they help your defenses.
Our bodies they clean, and our muscles they harden,
No wonder God grew them in the very first Garden!

When it comes to best food that our money can buy,
Some say it's hamburgers, pizzas, and pie.
But if you're like me, and good health is the question,
You can't beat the stuff in the ol' produce section.

WHY EAT FRUITS?

Fruits have a number of qualities that lend themselves to healthful eating. Three of these qualities and their positive effects follow.

Cleansing
According to nutritionist Ann Wigmore, fruits are on the average 90 percent liquid.[1] Their water is the most health-promoting fluid on planet earth. It serves to clean out our systems by flushing our cells, bathing our tissues, and stimulating the workings of our metabolic processes.

Satisfying
Nutritionist Harvey Diamond points out that "fruit contains all of the necessary nutrients required by your body for sustaining life. That includes glucose from carbohydrates for energy and vitamins, minerals, fatty acids, and amino acids for the building of protein."[2]

Not only do they satisfy many of our requirements for life, they also satisfy our sweet tooth with their natural sugars.

Energizing
"The digestion of food takes more body energy than any other function."[3] Fruit, however, is the only food that gives energy without taking it. Its natural sugars give our bodies an energy boost while at the same time requiring virtually no digestive energies from our bodies. Ripe, whole fruits and freshly made fruit juices (not bottled or frozen) are loaded with their own digestive enzymes which go to work quickly in our stomachs. Within thirty minutes or so, the nutrients in fruit have been released into the intestines for absorption.

WHY EAT VEGETABLES?

Vegetables, too, are essential to a healthy diet. We have listed some of vegetables' contributions to proper eating.

High in Vitamins and Minerals
In his classic book *Food Is Your Best Medicine*, Henry G. Bieler, M.D., points out that "a stalk of celery or a serving of fresh salad greens has more vitamins and minerals than a box of synthetic vitamin tablets."[4]

Another fact that will no doubt surprise you is that certain vegetables provide more milligrams of calcium per 3 ½-ounce portion than cow's milk! These include broccoli, mustard greens, watercress, turnip greens, kale, dandelion greens, collards, parsley, and kelp (a sea vegetable). So much for the theory that you must drink milk in order to have strong bones and healthy teeth!

High in Dietary Fiber
Both fruits and vegetables are excellent sources of dietary fiber. Dr. Norman Walker refers to it as the "intestinal broom." Without fiber in our diets, the kinds of foods we tend to eat most as Americans can "leave a coating of slime on the inner walls of the colon (large intestine) like plaster on a wall. In the course of time this coating may gradually increase its thickness until there is only a small hole through the center."[5] This is toxic waste that serves to gradually and continuously poison the entire body. Many health professionals consider a poorly functioning colon a fundamental cause of degenerative disease. The British Medical Society stated its position that "death begins in the colon."

High-fiber diets help to keep this condition from happening. (See "Plan 'Fast' Days" for more information on how to help keep your colon cleaned out.)

Packed with Anticancer Nutrients
The carrot is king of the "cabbage patch" when it comes to waging war on cancer. It is high in beta-carotene, a plant form of vitamin A. Certain members of the cruciferous wing of the vegetable family also have chemical properties that help to combat cancer. These include cabbage, broccoli, Brussels sprouts, kohlrabi, and cauliflower.[6]

Low in the Bad Stuff

Not only are fruits and vegetables low in fat and devoid of cholesterol, they're also low on the food chain. This means they will contain fewer contaminants from pesticides and other environmental toxins than the farm animals that eat them and store up concentrated amounts of pollutants in their flesh and fat. When you and I consume animal products . . . well, you see the progression.

WHY RAW?

The answer is simple—enzymes! Raw fruits and vegetables have them. Cooked don't.

So what are enzymes? "Catalysts," explains medical doctor Richard O. Brennan, "the essential biological catalysts that make life possible."[7] In fact, enzymes are a form of protein that initiate every biological cell or organ reaction that occurs in our bodies. Like a car without spark plugs, a body without enzymes is dead. "Without enzymes we would be a worthless pile of lifeless chemical substances—vitamins, minerals, protein, and water," observes nutritionist Ann Wigmore.[8] Medical researcher and author Carlson Wade refers to enzymes as "youth workers,"[9] a fitting description since enzymes serve to build, revitalize, and regenerate our cells and systems.

The most important function enzymes perform is the digestion and assimilation of nutrients from the food we eat. *Raw* fruits and vegetables are packed with health-promoting nutrients, whereas cooking destroys many of these. They are also loaded with their own digestive enzymes that help our body's enzyme force remove and utilize these nutrients. These built-in workmen in raw foods thus serve to enhance the quality and quantity of nutrient assimilation, while at the same time allowing our body to conserve its own enzyme energy and redirect it toward maintaining other systems.

Ann Wigmore observes, "Few withdrawals (cooked food) and large deposits (raw food) are the key. . . . If food enzymes do some of the work in the act of predigestion, the metabolic enzyme account can allot less activity to digestive enzymes, and have much more to give to the hundreds of enzyme systems that run the body."[10]

This conservation of enzyme energy is important. It's as if when we were formed in our mother's womb, God put a fixed supply of these "sparks of life" in our metabolic bank account. Depending upon the food we eat, cooked or raw, we are either shrinking or adding to that account.

Concerning this Dr. Brennan writes, "The enzyme content of organisms is depleted with increasing age . . . it is important that we recognize as early in life as possible that we must guard wisely this gift of health (our supply of enzymes) in order to insure maintenance of enzyme activity throughout our lifetime." He goes on to point out that "the emphasis on eating as many raw, uncooked foods as possible is of great significance."[11] Enzymes begin to die at 107 degrees Fahrenheit and are completely destroyed at 122 degrees Fahrenheit.[12]

WHY ORGANIC?

We hear a lot about organic foods these days—and with good reason. If you want to eat better foods, you should seriously consider "going organic." For the following reasons.

Minimized Exposure to Toxic Chemicals
Basically, organic produce is grown without the use of synthetic fertilizers and pesticides. More natural means for fertilizing are used, including composts, manure, untreated mineral rock powders, and nitrogen-fixed crops such as legumes. Organic pesticides, derived from plants, are used and have very little negative impact, if any, on soil, health, and the environment.[13]

Lest you think all this fuss over getting things "organic" is silly, here are a few important facts:

▶ In the United States, the use of pesticides has increased thirty-three-fold since it all began back in the 1940s.[14]

- Of the 350 "active" ingredients allowed in various pesticides, at least 70 are classified by the Environmental Protection Agency (EPA) as being potentially carcinogenic.[15] Most consumer-protection organizations believe this number is low.
- Of the 1,200 or so "inert" ingredients in pesticide products, more than 800 lack adequate data on toxicity. (Formulas are trade secrets. Manufacturers don't have to list inert ingredients on their labels.)[16] Of those that have been identified and tested, forty proved to be of toxic concern.[17]
- "In 1987 the EPA ranked pesticide residues in food 3rd in terms of cancer risk, of 31 problems under their jurisdiction."[18]

Maximized Nutrition

Unfortunately, the current "mainstream" methods of farming are wearing out our soils. In fact, we're actually losing much of our topsoil in this country because of current practices. It's estimated that 75 percent of it is now gone, most of this happening since the 1920s. "As a result, almost ⅓ of US cropland is showing a steady and serious decline in productivity."[19]

In organic farming, however, the main objective is to build healthy soils. Organic farmers feed the soil, not the plant. In so doing, they create an environment for plant growth that multiplies the nutritional values present in the produce.

KEY QUOTES

There is more and more acknowledgment by men of science that raw, uncooked food in the diet is indispensable to the highest degree of health.
Richard O. Brennan, D.O., M.D.
Coronary? Cancer? God's Answer: Prevent It!

Only whole natural foods can provide all the basic nutrients. . . . If one were to eat

*only cooked food or frozen food, he would develop
deficiency problems because certain nutrients
would not be supplied as needed.*
Alan H. Nittler, M.D.
A New Breed of Doctor

*Vegetables cost me my first husband, a woman remarked.
I hope my second husband will eat them.*
Author Unknown

*All the nutritional requirements that the human body has—
all the vitamins, minerals, proteins, amino acids, enzymes,
carbohydrates, and fatty acids that exist,
that the human body needs to survive—are to be found
in fruits and vegetables.*
Harvey and Marilyn Diamond
Fit for Life

HOW TO PUT MORE PRODUCE IN YOUR DIET

Much more could be said about why you should eat raw, organic fruits and vegetables, but hopefully I have given you just enough information to motivate you in that direction. Time now for a few practical how-to's that will help you build this healthy habit.

Buy Organic Produce

Find a store or co-op that offers certified organic produce. Health-food stores are becoming commonplace as more of us are paying attention to the link between diet and disease. The good ones will label each food product as to whether or not it is organically grown. Co-ops have also formed where members work one afternoon a week in exchange for lower prices on organic goods. Even regular supermarkets are getting into the act, stocking small supplies of organic produce to satisfy their customers who are asking. Add your voice.

If you simply can't find organic produce anywhere nearby,

here are some things you can do to help minimize your exposure to toxic chemicals:

- ▶ **Buy "in season."** Out-of-season produce is likely to be imported. Chances are greater that it will contain pesticides banned in the United States.
- ▶ **Wash your produce before eating.** One-fourth cup of hydrogen peroxide to a sink of water.
- ▶ **Peel your produce.** Peeling does completely remove surface pesticides and waxes, but you will also be losing fiber and nutrients. "As a general rule, peel produce if your diet is otherwise rich in fiber—especially produce that is obviously waxed, to remove the wax and any pesticides that might have been applied with it."[20]

Eat Fruit for Breakfast and Snacks

In the 1940s a scientist by the name of Are Waerland identified the fact that our bodies go through three distinct, yet sometimes overlapping, cycles during a twenty-four-hour period. These cycles are reflective of how our bodies metabolize food. In their book *Living Health*, Harvey and Marilyn Diamond define the cycles as follows:

Appropriation (eating and digestion)—
    noon to 8:00 p.m.
Assimilation (absorption and use)—
    8:00 p.m. to 4:00 a.m.
Elimination (of body wastes and food debris)—
    4:00 a.m. to noon[21]

These cycles are not mutually exclusive. One or more may be happening in the body at any one time. But one will always be predominant over the others, carrying out the primary task associated with the particular time period at hand.

Since breakfast falls between the hours of 4:00 a.m. and noon, a cycle when your body is working hard to rid itself of waste, eating a big breakfast is counterproductive. This is where fresh, raw fruit comes in. It is full of enzymes that make it the easiest food on the planet for your body to digest, it is saturated with natural sugars that get you going, it is loaded with vitamins and minerals to keep you strong, and it's packed with fiber to assist in the waste removal process. Many in the field of nutrition consider fresh, organic fruit the perfect food for breakfast. Since we're all biologically unique, our daily cycles will vary somewhat. Try eating fruit for breakfast for a week to see if you function better.

There is one rule about consuming fruit which must be followed. Eat it only on an empty stomach. The habit of following up a meal with a piece of fruit interferes with proper digestion. Fruit passes through the stomach so quickly that if it is held up by slower digesting foods, it begins to ferment. Yeast, also known as candida, thrives on fermentation and is a very unpleasant type of health condition to try to deal with. We all have a little yeast in our intestinal tracts, but we don't want to feed it by eating in such a way as to cause fermentation. Other than this one little rule, fruit is a great between-meal snack.

Eat Salads for Lunch and with Dinner
There are several cookbooks on the market that will help you with creative salad ideas. Be very careful about the kinds of dressings you use. Many are loaded with fat and sugar.

KEY QUESTIONS

Q. I want to eat more raw fruits and vegetables, but they always seem to go bad on me before I get around to eating them. What can I do to keep them fresh?

A. Here are a few tips that will help you not only keep your produce fresh, but ensure that you're getting maximum nutrients from them:

1. Store fruits and vegetables in plastic bags or airtight containers in the drawers of your refrigerator. These are usually colder and more humid than the rest of the refrigerated space.

2. Just before you plan to eat your produce, wash it in cold water using a nontoxic soap. Rinse thoroughly and pat dry.

3. Try to buy produce the size you need for one meal and use the whole thing. When you cut up or break apart a fruit or vegetable item, vitamins and enzymes immediately begin to be destroyed due to exposure to light and oxygen. It is therefore better to eat the whole thing at once than to save part of it in the refrigerator for another meal. For instance, Karen MacNeil notes in *The Book of Whole Foods: Nutrition and Cuisine* that "cucumbers lose 22% of their vitamin C when they're sliced. If sliced cucumbers are left for one hour, the loss jumps to 35%. If they're left for three hours, 49%."[22]

4. Perhaps the most obvious hint is to shop often for produce, perhaps every third day or so. Stocking up for a week at a time simply doesn't work. Buy often and eat often. That's the true secret to keeping your produce fresh and full of nutrients.

Q. What about steaming vegetables occasionally?

A. Raw is, of course, best as far as enzymes and nutrients are concerned. Lightly steaming is second best. Use just enough water under the steam basket to do the job without touching the vegetables. Steam them just enough to allow them to remain crisp. But again, don't give up raw for steamed. Steamed vegetables make a nice addition to a cooked meal, but keep your intake of raw produce going as well.

FURTHER READING

The Book of Whole Foods: Nutrition and Cuisine by Karen MacNeil (New York: Vintage Books, 1981). Separate chapters entitled "Vegetables" and "Fruits" contain excellent information on storage and preparation of these foods.

Coronary? Cancer? God's Answer: Prevent It! by Richard O. Brennan, D.O., M.D. (Irvine, CA: Harvest House,

1979). See chapter 7: "Magic Enzymes."

Everyday Cancer Risks and How to Avoid Them by Mary
Kerney Levenstein (Garden City Park, NY: Avery
Publishing Group, 1992). See chapter 11: "Pesticides in
Foods."

Food Enzymes, The Missing Link to Radiant Health by
Humbart Santillo, B.S., M.H. (Prescott, AZ: Hohm Press,
1987). A good resource for understanding enzymes.

*Helping Yourself with New Enzyme Catalyst Health
Secrets* by Carlson Wade (West Nyack, NY: Parker
Publishing Co., 1981). Perhaps a bit overstated, yet help-
ful in understanding the benefits of enzymes.

The Hippocrates Diet and Health Program by Ann
Wigmore (Wayne, NJ: Avery Publishing Group, 1984).
See chapter 3: "The Secret of Health" for enzyme
information.

Safe Food by Michael F. Jacobson, Ph.D., Lisa Y. Lefferts,
and Anne Witte Garland (Los Angeles: Living Planet
Press, 1991). See chapter 2: "Fruits, Vegetables, and
Grains" for information about pesticides.

8
BUILD COOKED MEALS AROUND STARCHES

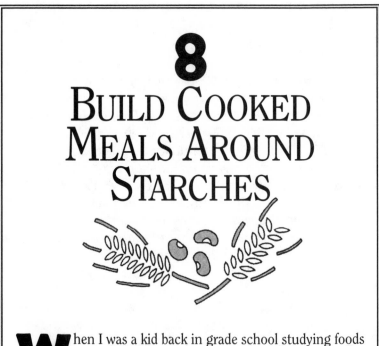

When I was a kid back in grade school studying foods in health class, my introduction to the term *starches* as a food category conjured up a rather negative image. With a shudder, I envisioned myself sitting down at the dinner table to a big aerosol spray can of laundry starch, the same sort of stuff my grandma used on shirt collars. Eeeeyyyuck!

Since those early days of "pioneering" my way through dangerous notions in the world of food science, I've come to better understand food starches. Referred to along with fruits and vegetables as *complex carbohydrates*, the starch family includes:

▶ *Whole grains*: brown rice, wheat berries, bulgur (cracked), millet, rye, triticale, barley, oats, corn, buckwheat, quinoa (pronounced kēn′ wä), amaranth
▶ *Legumes*:
  beans—pinto, pink, kidney, white, black, lima, mung, garbanzo, soy, azuki, navy, great northern, fava
  peas—green and yellow split, black-eyed, whole green
  lentils—green, red, brown

▶ *Roots*: white potatoes, sweet potatoes, yams, parsnips, taro, rutabaga

▶ *Squashes*: acorn, hubbard, banana, pumpkin, spaghetti, butternut

Instead of meat, these are the kinds of foods we ought to reach for when wanting to build a meal around something cooked.

WHY EAT STARCHES?

As we've already seen, the centerpiece of the standard American diet (SAD) is the ever-present slab of meat, more often than not loaded with saturated fat, always high in cholesterol, and always lacking any fiber.

Starches, on the other hand, bring to the plate a strong lineup of traits that far and away outdo meat as a star player on any cooked food menu.

MEAT	STARCHES
High fat	Low fat
Cholesterol	No cholesterol
No fiber	Loaded with fiber
Cancer promoting	Protective against cancer
Circulatory-disease promoting	Protective against fat and cholesterol deposits

There're no two ways about it. A vegetarian diet is clearly health promoting, while a meat-based diet clearly is not. Diets built around starches, fruits, and vegetables provide the best fuel for your body.

KEY QUOTES

Nutritional research done over the past fifty years confirms not only the adequacy of a starch-centered diet supplemented with fresh fruits and vegetables,

but also its superiority. Unlike meat that is high in protein
and fat, and has no fiber, a plant-based diet
provides "just the right amounts of protein, essential fat,
fiber, water, vitamins, and minerals."
John A. McDougall, M.D.
The McDougall Plan

Carbohydrates in the form of starch have been
the ideal source of human energy for centuries.
A human's large brain requires
a high glucose diet (found in starch), which also provides
warmth and fuel.
Gordon S. Tessler, Ph.D.
Lazy Man's Guide to Better Nutrition

Foods high in complex carbohydrates—grains, vegetables,
and fruits—are the best foods you can eat.
Nathan Pritikin, scientist
The Pritikin Program for Diet and Exercise

The average age (longevity) of a meat eater is 63.
I am on the verge of 85 and still work as hard as ever.
I have lived quite long enough and I am trying to die; but I
simply cannot do it. A single beef-steak would finish me,
but I cannot bring myself to swallow it. I am oppressed
with a dread of living forever.
This is the only disadvantage to vegetarianism.
George Bernard Shaw (1856–1950)

BREAD, THE STAFF OF LIFE!

Man does not live by bread alone, but life would sure be a bum-
mer without it. If you enjoy homemade bread as much as we
do, perhaps you will appreciate a few hints about how to ensure
its highest level of nutrition.

Buying sacks of whole-grain flour at your local grocery store
is probably a mistake. Once grain has been milled, oxidation of

the oil in it commences rapidly, and the flour can become rancid within a week. Rancid food ingredients are counterproductive to good health. There is no way of telling when supermarket-sold flour was milled, how long it sat in a warehouse, and how long it's been sitting on the grocer's shelf.

A better choice would be to purchase bread at the health-food store or a shop that specializes in baking organic, whole-grain breads. Be sure you are getting 100 percent whole-grain bread. Find out also if the baker uses freshly milled flour, preferably made from organically grown grain.

Perhaps you can find a local source of freshly milled grain to purchase for use in making your own bread at home. If so, keep it in an airtight container in the freezer compartment of your refrigerator, away from light, heat, and oxygen. These elements speed spoilage. Plan to use it up within a few weeks.

Ultimately, you ought to consider investing in your own grain mill. Anne and I have one in our garage. They're relatively small machines, no bigger than a bread box, and run about $150.00. If that's beyond your means, perhaps you could go in with a friend or two, sharing the machine. (We buy our grain—wheat, oats, and rice—in fifty-pound bags from a friend who runs a grain business out of her garage. Health-food stores usually have bins full of fresh grains; bakeries sometimes sell grains bulk.)

"BEAN, BEANS, THE MUSICAL FRUIT"

Remember that one from your childhood? "The more you eat the more you'll toot." That's the problem for most of us with beans—and in fact the larger category of whole foods called legumes, of which beans are a part. We love them, but they don't love us, causing bloating and gas. Actually, the problem many of us experience with legumes is due to their complex sugars (otherwise known as oligosaccharides), "which arrive intact in the large intestine and are not easily broken down by enzymes."[1]

There are some things you can do to help make legumes a more pleasing part of your cuisine.

1. Try soaking your legumes overnight in a pot of water. Discard this water and refill with fresh before cooking. You lose some of the nutrients, but the soaking also removes some of the complex sugars, making your legumes more digestible and their remaining nutrients more readily utilized.
2. Another approach you might try is to boil your legumes for thirty minutes to an hour, then discard that water. Fill again with fresh water, and continue to boil.
3. Always cook legumes thoroughly. The softer they are, the more easily digested.
4. Don't salt legumes before or during cooking. This makes their skins tougher and harder to digest.
5. Emphasize split peas and lentils. These are usually more readily digested than other legumes, and they don't need to be soaked.
6. Consider taking a digestive enzyme supplement when you eat legumes. We keep a supply of them in our own kitchen cabinet for just such a purpose.

MENUS

Here are a few meal ideas that we enjoy around our house that seat starches at the "head of the table." Give them a try. See what you like. Be creative and come up with more.

▶ Baked Beans and Garden Salad
▶ Corn Bread and Antipasto (tomatoes, onions, olives, garbanzo beans, artichoke hearts, avocado with Italian dressing)
▶ Steamed Green Peppers (stuffed with brown rice and veggie mix or whole-grain stuffing)
▶ Pita Pockets (pita bread stuffed with spinach salad)
▶ Baked Acorn Squash and Broccoli/Cauliflower Vinaigrette (vinegar and oil)
▶ Cold Pasta Salad (with lots of veggies and Italian dressing)

- ▶ Baked Potato Bar (Cover baked potatoes with your choice of ingredients—tomato, broccoli, onion, olives, sunflower seeds, whole-grain bread crumbs, cauliflower, avocado, etc.)
- ▶ Spaghetti Squash with Tomato Sauce and Tossed Salad
- ▶ Red Lentil Soup with Carrot Sticks and Whole-Wheat Rolls
- ▶ Whole-Wheat Tortillas (stuffed with beans, tomatoes, lettuce, olives, etc.)
- ▶ Tom Burgers (whole-wheat buns, barbecued onions, tomato, sprouts, pickles, avocado)
- ▶ Brown Rice with Steamed Veggies

FURTHER READING

Amazing Grains by Joanne Saltzman (Tiburon, CA: H. J. Kramer, 1990). Creating vegetarian main dishes with whole grains.

The American Vegetarian Cookbook by Marilyn Diamond (New York: Warner Books, 1990).

The Book of Whole Foods by Karen MacNeil (New York: Vintage Books, 1981). See "Carbohydrates," pages 33-35.

Jane Brody's Nutrition Book by Jane Brody (New York: Bantam Books, 1984). See chapter 5: "Carbohydrates Have Gotten a Bad Press."

9
CUT BACK ON REFINED SUGARS

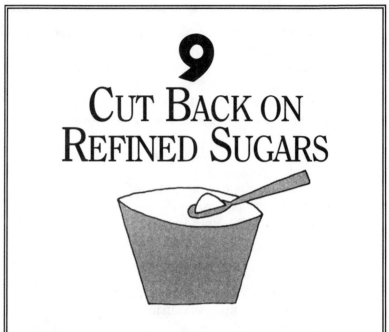

Many doctors, nutritionists, and researchers consider refined sugar a major nemesis of American health. Nevertheless, sugar is, hands down, America's number one food additive. Would you believe that we consume ten times more of it than we do all the other 2,600 or so food additives put together?! The one exception is salt, but even it runs a very distant second.[1]

Every year the typical American consumes between 120 and 150 pounds of refined sugar.[2] That translates to over one-third of a pound a day, 600-plus calories of teeth-rotting, health-destroying sweetness. Sort of a contradiction in terms.

Even if you don't eat sweets, the amount of refined sugar you may be consuming would no doubt shock you. Over two-thirds of the refined sugar used in this country is added to manufactured food products. In other words, it's hidden in many of the things we buy at the supermarket. For instance, did you know that a tablespoon of ketchup contains a full teaspoon of sugar?[3] Stuff like breads, soups, cereals, cured meats, hot dogs, lunch meat, salad dressings, spaghetti sauce, crackers, mayonnaise, peanut butter, pickles, frozen pizza, canned fruits and vegetables, tomato juice, and a host of other products all contain sugar. This doesn't even take into account the obvious sugary products like candies, cakes, ice cream, cookies, doughnuts, and soda pop.

Even if you are careful about reading labels, it's difficult to tell just how much refined sugar you're actually getting. It comes in many different forms, several of which might be contained in a single product. Terms like *sucrose, fructose, glucose, maltose,* and *lactose* may mean something to a scientist (or "scientose"), but how are average laypeople supposed to understand what they're putting into their mouths?

And what about all those other products that we use to sweeten our food? Are molasses, maple syrup, corn syrup, and honey just as bad for your health as white sugar?

Obviously, there are many questions that arise in any discussion about sugars and sweeteners. Let's pick off a few and see if we can't get some understanding.

WHAT ARE THE VARIOUS FORMS OF SUGARS?

Sucrose
More commonly known as white, refined table sugar, it comes from sugar cane, sugar beets, and sugar maples, and is the most widely used form of sugar. The following is a list of products in the sucrose family:[4]

White sugar	99.9 percent sucrose
Turbinado sugar	99 percent sucrose
Brown sugar	96 percent sucrose
Maple sugar	95-98 percent sucrose
Maple syrup	65 percent sucrose
Molasses	50-70 percent sucrose

Fructose
Also known as levulose, fructose is found naturally in fruits and honey. It can also be commercially refined from corn, sugar beets, and sugar cane. Currently, the most popular form of refined

fructose is corn syrup, which is added to hundreds of products. Since it is about 70 percent sweeter than sucrose,[5] many food manufacturers now use refined fructose to replace refined sucrose in their products—same sweetness, fewer calories.

Maltose

This form of sugar results from "malting" certain grains together with natural enzymes. Two of the most popular forms are barley malt and brown rice syrup. Barley malt is made by sprouting barley, drying it, then mixing it with water and cooking it into a syrup. Brown rice syrup is made by adding dried sprouted barley to cooked rice. After the rice is cultured, it is strained and cooked to produce a syrup. Maltose is about one-third as sweet as sucrose.[6]

Glucose

Also known as dextrose, glucose is found naturally in fruit, honey, carob, and corn, or may also be found in refined form. It is about two-thirds as sweet as sucrose.[7] Glucose is also the form that all sugars are broken down to by our bodies to be utilized for energy.

(Special note: Lactose is the form of sugar found in milk. Another form of milk sugar is called galactose. These are not consumed in sugar form, but as part of milk products. Therefore, they are not usually considered food additives.)

WHICH SUGARS ARE BETTER FOR US?

As far as nutritional benefit to our bodies, all simple sugars are empty calories—about four per gram. As regards their impact upon our bodies, sucrose is the worst. It demands the production of insulin by our pancreas, causes significant fluctuation in blood-sugar levels, and robs nutrients from various stores in our bodies in order to be digested.

The myth of "quick energy" that accompanies refined sugar products such as candy bars and other sweets that are high in sucrose (white sugar) is destroyed by the reality that a temporary "sugar high" from this form of sugar is followed quickly by the "sugar blues."

The following is a list of generally accepted substitutes for sucrose. Although no sweetener is without problems, these seem to have less negative impact upon the body.

- ▶ *Fruit juice*—Because it is fructose, it causes less of a rise in blood-sugar levels than sucrose. Fructose sugars don't require insulin. They are metabolized in our liver rather than our small intestine, as is sucrose. They are also absorbed more slowly into our bloodstream than sucrose.
- ▶ *Date sugar*—Ground-up dates. The sugar in dates is predominantly fructose.
- ▶ *Maltose*—A complex natural sugar that requires some breaking down into simple sugars in our bodies. It has no sucrose in it. Like fructose, maltose is metabolized by enzymes that do not require insulin. No fluctuations in blood-sugar levels are caused by maltose. Amasake (a sweet pudding-like substance made from cultured brown rice), barley malt, and brown rice syrup are examples of maltose.
- ▶ *Sucanat*—This product is made by squeezing the juice from sugar cane, then evaporating the water through a special process. What's left is a substitute for white refined sugar that contains vitamins, minerals, and trace elements—all of which refined sugar does not.
- ▶ *FruitSource*—Derived from a mixture of fruit and grains, it contains both simple and complex carbohydrates as well as small amounts of proteins, fats, vitamins, and minerals.
- ▶ *Amasake*—A whole-grain pudding-like sweetener made by adding fermented brown rice to cooked rice.
- ▶ *Honey*—It rots teeth faster than sucrose,[8] and because it is a simple sugar it can cause fluctuations in blood-sugar levels.[9] The more fructose is in it, however, the less significant the blood-sugar changes. Different types

of honey have different types of sugar, depending upon the crops the bees drew pollen from. For instance, clover honey is 60 percent sucrose, which would tend to cause more significant blood-sugar changes than orange blossom honey, which is 70 percent fructose.[10] Use only raw, unfiltered honey, although most honey is heated to some degree during bottling. If you can, buy it from a farmer or roadside stand where less processing is likely to have taken place. The more cloudy it is, the better. And if it crystallizes, that's a sign that it's had less destructive heat applied to it. Honeys produced in your own locale tend to operate in your body as antiallergens, helping you counteract the effects of local allergy-producing substances.[11]

▶ *Maple syrup*—It does contain about 65 percent sucrose. Compared to white sugar, however, its negative impact upon blood-sugar levels is less.

▶ *Unsulfured blackstrap molasses*—Molasses is the liquid that remains after sucrose is refined from sugar cane or sugar beets. It has the same energy-exhausting effect on the body as white sugar, although somewhat less intense. It can also contain concentrated amounts of the stuff that was on the sugar cane or beets, like pesticides and environmental toxins. If sulfur was involved in processing out the sucrose, traces of this can remain as well.[12] Even with all of this potentially stacked against it, blackstrap molasses is recommended by some as a viable substitute for white sugar. It does contain nutrients (calcium, iron, potassium, and B vitamins) that have been refined out of white sugar. The darker the molasses, the more nutritious, with blackstrap being the best.[13]

WHAT DO REFINED SUGARS DO TO THE BODY?

Refined sugars have a negative effect on the body, the details of which are explored below.

Tooth Decay

The bacteria in our mouths use sugar in our diet to form substances that cause tooth decay. These include a gummy material called glucan that helps the bacteria stick to our teeth, plus acids that corrode the protective enamel.

Obesity

Sugars are no more fattening than starch or protein. The problem is that you can pack a lot of sugar calories into a small amount of food. If our diets contain a lot of sugary foods, we tend to overconsume calories long before our stomachs are full. This overconsumption of sugar not only leads to becoming overweight, but the potential onset of diabetes becomes multiplied.

Hypoglycemia

This is a condition in which the pancreas overproduces insulin to deal with an influx of sugar and thus lowers blood-sugar levels (which is true for many of us), but the mechanism by which the resulting low blood sugar is restored to balance is not working properly. This leaves the individual in a low-blood-sugar or hypoglycemic state. Often he or she will consume more sugar to help restore his or her system, which in turn leads to further problems.[14]

Diabetes

"There is no doubt," writes David Reuben, M.D., "that diabetes mellitus—otherwise known as 'sugar diabetes'—is caused by excessive consumption of refined sugar."[15]

The simple truth is that refined sugars, also known as simple sugars, break down too quickly into glucose in our small intestine and are too rapidly absorbed into our bloodstream, causing a condition known as hyperglycemia, or what is often referred to as a "sugar high."

It's the job of our pancreas to control blood-sugar levels by producing insulin, a substance which transports glucose to our cells for energy, and any excess to our livers for storage as glycogen. With an influx of rapidly absorbed simple sugars, the pancreas overproduces insulin to protect our brain and other vital organs from sugar overdose. This rapid overproduction of insulin, which is triggered by refined sugar, soon results in too much sugar being removed from the blood. The result is a low-blood-sugar condition known as hypoglycemia—also referred to as the "sugar blues." At this point, our adrenal glands secrete a hormone that changes the stored glycogen into glucose to raise our blood-sugar levels again. Over time, this up and down roller coaster of metabolic needs due to the fluctuations of sugar ingestion leads to overtaxed, worn-out adrenal glands, liver, and pancreas.

"If your pancreas is forced to overproduce insulin for an extended period of time (20-30 years)," observes Dr. Gordon Tessler, "you run the risk of damaging the insulin producing mechanism."[16] Diabetes, the third-leading disease in this country behind heart disease and cancer, is in many cases due to a pancreas that is not producing enough insulin, having been exhausted by long-time consumption of simple or refined sugars.

"Raw Nerves," Osteoporosis, and Arthritis

All sugar eaten, whether natural or refined, requires B-complex vitamins, calcium, and magnesium for digestion. Complex carbohydrates, such as fruits, vegetables, and starches, contain enough of these nutrients to assist our bodies in their own digestion. However, the simple and refined sugars do not. Therefore, our bodies must call upon their stores of these nutrients in order to deal with this kind of sugar. B-complex is stolen from the nervous system, and calcium and magnesium are robbed from the bones and teeth. "Consequently," observes Dr. Tessler, "refined sugar 'rips you off' of these needed nutrients, resulting in 'raw' nerves."[17]

With a steady loss of calcium and magnesium from our bones and teeth, osteoporosis is a likely outcome—a dangerous softening of the bones and skeletal structure. And these released minerals float around in our bodies and they end up in part in our joints where they accumulate, a condition known as arthritis.

Impaired Immune System Functioning
The following chart shows what refined sugar can do to the effectiveness of our white blood cells, those members of our immune system that eat up foreign invaders, and in fact seek out and destroy our own cells that have become cancerous.

EFFECT OF REFINED SUGAR ON WHITE BLOOD CELL ACTIVITY[18]		
Amount Refined Sugar Consumed	Number of Bacteria a WBC Can Destroy in ½ Hour	Decrease in Immunity
No sugar	14	0%
6 teaspoons = 8 oz. of soft drink	10	25%
12 teaspoons = frosted brownie	5.5	60%
18 teaspoons = apple pie à la mode	2	85%
24 teaspoons = banana split	1	92%
Uncontrolled Diabetic	1	92%

(Special Note: A 12-ounce can of soda contains 9 teaspoons of sugar. An 8-ounce serving of fruit-flavored yoghurt contains almost as much.)[19]

Candida Albicans
Often referred to simply as candida, this organism is a normal fungus (yeast) that lives in our bodies. It normally takes up residence in our intestinal tract, but can get into our circulatory system. No one really knows what good it does our bodies, if any. Perhaps the only reason it's there is to help the decaying process of changing our bodies back into dust when we die.

If our blood chemistry is in good order and our immune system is strong, candida is kept in check. However, if these systems are not up to par, the fungus begins to overgrow our bodies. In his book *The Yeast Connection*, William G. Crook, M.D., puts forth an extensive list of symptoms indicating possible yeast overgrowth. Among them are fatigue, lethargy, depression, irritability, headaches, inability to concentrate, inappropriate drowsiness, muscle weakness and numbing, recurrent vaginal or urinary tract infections, athlete's foot, jock itch, persistent digestive distresses (heartburn, indigestion, constipation, etc.), swollen joints, nasal congestion, recurrent sore throats, and more.[20]

As was already pointed out, a steady intake of refined sugar in our diets can weaken the effectiveness of our immune systems, thus allowing candida to multiply. This, plus the fact that yeast feeds on sugar, makes refined sugar a real no-no.

And Much, Much More

This list could go on and on. In fact, Nancy Appleton, Ph.D., author of *Lick the Sugar Habit*, lists the following potential consequences of long-term consumption of refined sugars: hypoglycemia, diabetes, constipation, stomach or intestinal gas, arthritis, asthma, headaches, psoriasis, cancer, osteoporosis, heart disease, obesity, candida albicans, tooth decay, multiple sclerosis, inflammatory bowel disease, canker sores, gallstones, and cystic fibrosis.[21]

KEY QUOTES

*The major addiction problem in the United States and,
to a large extent, in the Western world, has nothing to do
with opiates, uppers or downers,
or even alcohol or tobacco.
The number one addiction today is sugar.*
Harold W. Harper, M.D.
How You Can Beat the Killer Diseases

*If only a fraction of what is already known
about the effects of sugar were to be revealed
in relation to any other material*

used as a food additive,
that material would promptly be banned.
John Yudkin
Physician Biochemist and Emeritus Professor
of Nutrition at London University

Refined sugar is a thief.
Gordon S. Tessler, Ph.D.
Lazy Person's Guide to Better Nutrition

The white crystalline powder called sugar has caused
the human race more suffering and more agonizing death
than the white crystalline powder called cocaine.
David Reuben, M.D.
Everything You Always Wanted to Know About Nutrition

TIPS ON CUTTING DOWN ON REFINED SUGAR

Don't Buy "Sweets"
Stay out of the candy aisle at the grocery store. Steer clear of the pastry section. Avoid the dairy cases. When it comes to spending your hard-earned money on sugar, "just say no"!

Rid Your Kitchen of Refined Sugar
Go through your refrigerator and cabinets, reading labels. If you find anything with these words on it, throw it out immediately: sucrose, fructose (obviously the commercially refined kind), glucose, maltose, lactose, galactose, cane syrup, corn syrup, corn sugar, invert sugar, dextrose, or anything else that smacks of refined sugar.

But all that food from my kitchen will be wasted, you're saying. "I know you're tempted to give it to poor people," writes Dr. David Reuben of what you'll find in your kitchen, "but don't do it unless you have something against poor people. And above all, don't give it to the dog. For one thing, the overrefined junk you're getting rid of probably doesn't meet the US Department of Agriculture standards for animal feed. It could get you in trouble."[22]

Keep tossing until your kitchen is completely free from refined sugar. "Then if you need a 'fix,'" says Dr. Nancy Appleton, "you will have to drive to the store to feed your habit. This will give you time to think, and maybe you'll change your mind. If not, buy only enough to satisfy your craving. Don't buy any more than you can eat at the moment. Buy the smallest size of whatever it is you crave, and throw out what you don't eat. Better wasted outside the body than inside."[23]

Eat Lots of Complex Carbohydrates

Build your daily diet around an abundance of fruits, vegetables, and starches. These foods contain sugars that need breaking down before they enter your bloodstream. They keep your blood-sugar level on an even keel, not the up and down "yo-yo" effect of sweets made with refined sugar—sugar highs and sugar lows. As your blood-sugar level stabilizes, you will find yourself craving refined sugar products less and less. Your body simply doesn't need that instant sugar energy.

Examine the Stressors in Your Life

Many of us turn to food, especially sweets, for a sense of psychological comfort. I know that for me, if I'm frustrated, frightened, or angry, one of the ways I'm always tempted to deal with it is to lose myself in a Snickers bar. But if I do, I'm not only still frustrated, frightened, or angry, but I've added to my inner turmoil by being mad at myself for what I've just done to my body.

Next time you find yourself reaching for the Coke Classic or a Hershey's bar, stop and ask yourself why. Analyze the situation. Are you craving sugar, something you know is bad for your health, as a pacifier? A kind of appeasement for something that's going on outside your body? Try to identify those things that trigger your cravings for sugar and make every effort to control them.

KEY QUESTION

Q. If I'm trying to fight off a yeast overgrowth (candida), I know that I should avoid refined sugar. Should I also avoid fruit?

A. The best answer I can give to this question is that the field is split. There are professionals like John W. Rippon, Ph.D., (an authority on yeasts and molds) of the University of Chicago, who say yes.

Rippon: "Yeasts thrive on the simple carbohydrates. These include cane sugar, beet sugar, honey, corn syrup, maple syrup and molasses. In addition, eating fruits promotes yeast growth. Here's why. Fruits are loaded with fructose. In spite of their fiber content, fruits are readily converted to fructose and other simple sugars in the intestinal tract, thereby encouraging the growth of Candida Albicans."[24]

On the other hand, there are nutritionists and natural hygienists in the camp that Harvey and Marilyn Diamond represent who say no, it is not necessary to give up on fruit. The only precaution is the one that applies to anyone eating fruit—consume it alone and on an empty stomach.

Diamond: "If you have the Candida organism in your body, and almost everyone has, then be careful of fruit or anything else that can ferment in the body. The only way fruit can aggravate a Candida infection is if it is eaten incorrectly. When fresh fruit is eaten alone and on an empty stomach, it will *not* ferment! This is the key. When you eat cooked fruit or eat fruit with other foods, it spoils and ferments in the stomach. The Candida yeast proliferates on fermentable foods—carbohydrates. By consuming only fresh fruit when the stomach is entirely empty, there is no possibility of fermentation from bacteria or yeast."[25]

Perhaps a balance between these two opinions is represented by William Crook, M.D., previously mentioned as author of *The Yeast Connection*. He observes, "Some of my patients with yeast-connected illness tolerate complex carbohydrates, including apples, bananas and pineapple. If you are such a person, Karen Barkie's cookbook *Sweet and Sugar Free* (St. Martin's Press, New York, NY) should interest you. It's full of recipes for sugar-free, fruit-sweetened foods. Other of my patients develop symptoms when they eat fruits."[26]

The point is, if you're battling a yeast overgrowth, do some experimenting to see what effect fruit has on it in your own body.

FURTHER READING

The Book of Whole Foods: Nutrition and Cuisine by Karen MacNeil (New York: Vintage Books, 1981). See "Sugars and Sweeteners," pages 301-315.

Everything You Always Wanted to Know About Nutrition by David Reuben, M.D. (New York: Simon and Schuster, 1978). See chapter 10: "Sugar."

Jane Brody's Nutrition Book by Jane Brody (New York: Bantam Books, 1981). See chapter 6: "Sugar: Is Our Sweet Tooth Killing Us?"

Lazy Person's Guide to Better Nutrition by Gordon S. Tessler, Ph.D. (San Diego, CA: Better Health Publishers, 1984). See chapter 8: "Sugar: Friend or Foe?"

Lick the Sugar Habit by Nancy Appleton, Ph.D. (Garden City Park, NY: Avery Publishing Group, 1988).

Living Well by Dale and Kathy Martin (Brentwood, TN: Wolgemuth and Hyatt, 1988). See chapter 4: "The Rush to Diabetes."

Sugar Blues by William Dufty (New York: Warner Books, 1975).

The Yeast Connection by William G. Crook, M.D. (Jackson, TN: Professional Books, 1985).

10
CUT BACK ON SALT

Everybody needs some salt in his or her diet. Sodium is a vital mineral for health. It is primarily responsible for regulating the balance of water and dissolved substances outside our cells in our body fluids. Its counterpart, potassium, regulates fluids on the inside of our cells. Along with calcium and magnesium, these four minerals plus water form what is referred to as the "electrolyte soup" that bathes the interior of our bodies.[1]

WHY REDUCE SALT CONSUMPTION?

Although our bodies need salt, are we getting too much? The average American consumes three to five teaspoons of salt each day (7,000–10,000 milligrams).[2] The actual physiological requirement—220 milligrams a day—is only one-tenth of a teaspoon.[3] Even the RDA, which many health professionals believe to be exceedingly liberal concerning salt, suggests that a safe level of intake for an adult not exceed 3,300 milligrams. This translates to 1 3/5 teaspoons. Those who know nutrition are telling us we need to cut back. There are two primary reasons why.

Hypertension (High Blood Pressure)

Hypertension is a life-threatening disease. Often referred to as the "silent killer," it may exist for fifteen to twenty years without outward signs or symptoms, until one day, seemingly out of the blue, a crisis occurs. Hypertension has nothing to do with being hyper or tense, but with the pressure at which blood flows through your arteries. Excessive levels of salt in one's diet can contribute to this disease. Sodium draws water from the artery wall into the bloodstream, causing the artery to constrict while at the same time increasing fluid volume and pressure. The constant overload of salt in the typical American diet can mean consistently higher blood pressures. The more pressure, the greater the possibility of trouble.

High blood pressure has the potential to lead to a number of circulatory crises including kidney disease, heart attacks, and strokes. In Japan, where salt consumption is higher than any other place on earth, cerebral hemorrhages (strokes) are the leading cause of death.

Estimates are that as many as 60 million Americans have high blood pressure.[4] That's one out of every four of us. According to Julian Whitaker, M.D., author of the book *Reversing Health Risks*, anything above 140/90 represents high blood pressure.[5] In fact, John McDougall, M.D., suggests that an optimal blood pressure to shoot for is 110/70 or less.[6]

Treating high blood pressure has become big business for the medical community. According to Dr. McDougall, it has become the nation's leading reason for office visits to doctors and represents the number one health problem for which prescriptions are written. He notes that "each year Americans make about 25 million visits to their doctors to see about high blood pressure, and drugs are prescribed in 89 percent of those cases."[7]

Obviously, there are more natural and healthier means to deal with high blood pressure than to take drugs. Reducing salt in the diet is one. So is getting the right ratio of potassium to sodium. Eating more fruits and vegetables—potassium-rich foods—often helps to reduce high blood pressure.

The standard American diet is high in animal products (meat and dairy), which are naturally high in sodium. Medical writer Jane Brody observes, "Vegetarians, who generally consume a low-sodium, high-potassium diet, tend to have considerably lower blood pressure than other Americans their age."[8]

Another important part of the overall strategy to lower blood pressure is to lose weight. A leaner, trimmer you makes it easier for your heart to pump blood through the miles of blood vessels in your body.

Salt reduction, then, isn't the only tool in your toolbox to help you lower your blood pressure if it's high. It is, however, the tool recommended first by most doctors. Neal D. Barnard, M.D., writes in his book *The Power of the Plate*, "For everyone with high blood pressure, reduction in salt intake is a first step that your doctor will recommend. Leaving the salt shaker on the shelf helps reduce blood pressure."[9]

Hypersensitivity to Stress
There is a growing body of evidence that excess salt in the diet leads to an increased sensitivity to the stresses of life. Dr. Gordon Tessler observes that "Salt increases the number of brain-cell receptors for norepinephrine, the nervous system hormone that prepares the body for 'fight' or 'flight' in dangerous situations. Norepinephrine sends messages from the brain to the heart (heart pumps faster), the digestive system (all organs stop digestion), and the blood vessels (vessels constrict). With more norepinephrine produced because of salt overconsumption, a person becomes increasingly nervous and edgy."[10]

Additional Reasons
High sodium intake has also been found to interfere with the body's ability to remove fats from the bloodstream. It also is involved in kidney problems, water retention, cardiovascular disease, and possibly stomach cancer and migraine headaches.[11]

KEY QUOTES

*Common sense tells even the uninitiated
that it is wise to limit salt intake.
Indeed, if salt were a new food additive,
it is doubtful that it would be classified
as safe and certainly not at the level
most of us consume.*
Dr. Mark Hegsted
Head of the Human Nutrition Center
of the U.S. Department of Agriculture

*That salt-seeking instinct
may mean our own demise.*
Patrick Quillin, Ph.D., R.D.
Healing Nutrients

*It's clear that salt appetite is determined by early dietary
habits and has no relationship to salt need.*
Lot B. Page, M.D.

When it comes to salt, shake the habit!
Gordon S. Tessler, Ph.D.
Lazy Person's Guide to Better Nutrition

TIPS ON CUTTING BACK

1. *Cut back on food with visible salt*—potato chips, pretzels, corn chips, popcorn, crackers, shoestring potatoes, etc.

2. *Cut back on meat and dairy products.* Besides being naturally high in sodium, salt is added to many processed-meat and dairy products. These include cheese, butter, and processed meats. If you haven't already read the earlier chapters on meat and dairy, do so.

3. *Cut back on preserved or fermented foods*—pickles, sauerkraut, olives, soy sauce, etc.

4. *Eliminate canned foods, and replace with fresh or frozen.*

"Nearly ⅔'s of the salt in the American diet is consumed in processed foods."[12] For instance:

- ▶ 3 ½ ounces of fresh peas = 2 milligrams of sodium, while same amount of canned peas = 236 milligrams
- ▶ Six fresh spears of asparagus = 4 milligrams of sodium, while same amount of canned asparagus = 410 milligrams

5. *Read labels.* If you must buy processed foods, be sure to choose "low sodium" or "salt free." You'll be surprised at where you'll find hidden sources of sodium.[13]

- ▶ One ounce of Kellogg's Corn Flakes has nearly twice the amount of sodium as one ounce of Planters Cocktail Peanuts, 260 milligrams versus 132.
- ▶ Two slices of Pepperidge Farm White Bread have more sodium than a one-ounce bag of Lay's Potato Chips, 234 milligrams versus 191.
- ▶ ½ cup of prepared Jell-O Chocolate Flavor Instant Pudding and Pie Filling has more sodium than three slices of Oscar Mayer Sugar-cured Bacon, 404 milligrams versus 302.
- ▶ ½ cup of cottage cheese has as much sodium as thirty-two potato chips.

6. Cut back on soft drinks. Carbonated drinks contain bicarbonate of soda (sodium bicarbonate).

Buy a juicer and make your own fruit and vegetable juices, or drink purified water. According to Dr. Gordon Tessler, there's too much sodium in regular tap water to make it a healthy alternative.[14]

7. Use salt alternatives. The following are some generally accepted products used as salt alternatives:

- ▶ Quick Sip—a substitute for soy sauce
- ▶ Vegetable Broth Seasoning—a saltlike powder seasoning
- ▶ Vegit—an herb-based powder seasoning
- ▶ Spike (the salt-free variety)—a mixture of a variety of vegetables and herbs
- ▶ Braggs Liquid Aminos—a concoction of amino acids

made from soybeans that render a salty taste

8. Develop a taste for other spices. Empty your salt shakers and fill them with other flavorings. There are a host of herbs and spices that are available to add zest and interest to your foods. Experiment with different ones to find your favorites. Try allspice, basil, cayenne, chili powder, curry, dill, fennel, garlic, ginger root, lemon juice, lime juice, thyme, turmeric, and many, many others.

KEY QUESTIONS

Q. Is sea salt better than regular salt?

A. Because of government standards, they must both contain at least 97.5 percent sodium chloride. The difference between land-mined salt and sea salt taken from oceans by a process of evaporation is primarily the mineral content. Sea salt contains more. In most cases not a whole lot more, but enough for many nutritionists to suggest a switch to sea salt.

Q. If I go vegetarian and also quit using salt, won't I be in danger of getting too little sodium in my diet?

A. Gordon Tessler, Ph.D.: "There is enough natural salt in a wholesome diet of grains, seeds, nuts, vegetables and fruits to satisfy the adult daily sodium requirement."[15]

FURTHER READING

Everything You Always Wanted to Know About Nutrition by David Reuben, M.D. (New York: Simon and Schuster, 1978). See chapter 5: "Trace Elements."

Healing Nutrients by Patrick Quillin, Ph.D., R.D. (Chicago: Contemporary Books, 1987). See "Calcium, Magnesium, Sodium, and Potassium," pages 95-101.

Jane Brody's Nutrition Book by Jane Brody (New York: Bantam Books, 1981). See chapter 10: "Salt: Is the Pillar About to Collapse?"

Lazy Person's Guide to Better Nutrition by Gordon S. Tessler, Ph.D. (San Diego, CA: Better Health Publishers,

1984). See chapter 7: "Salt: Shake the Habit."
McDougall's Medicine: A Challenging Second Opinion by
John A. McDougall, M.D. (Piscataway, NJ: New Century
Publishers, 1985). See chapter 6: "Hypertension."

11
CHOOSE HEALTH-PROMOTING SNACKS

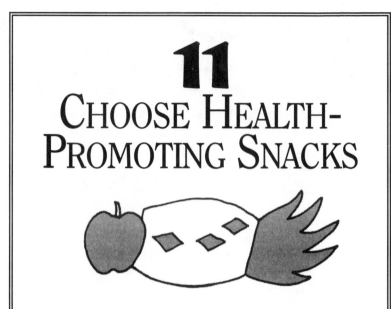

Americans are notorious for being "junk-food junkies." The manufacturing of junk-food products (pseudo-foods) that feed our habit has become the largest portion of the $416-billion-a-year food industry.[1]

Much of it is the stuff we reach for when we want a snack. Every day in the United States, thousands of us plunk a collective mountain of change into an untold number of vending machines from which we hope to draw some in between-meal pleasure. Clink, clink, clink, whirrrr, thunk—out drops a handful of something that is mostly sugar, perhaps some fat, perhaps some refined flour, perhaps some salt, perhaps some caffeine.

In the end, it's nothing but empty calories. For all the good it does our bodies, we might just as well eat the wrapper or the can.

The negative effects of junk-food snacks on our health wipe out the positive effects of health-promoting foods at mealtimes. Therefore, from now on when you want a snack, make it a healthy one.

BE PREPARED!

Snacking is not the problem in the American diet. The snacks are the problem. Preparation is *the* key to having healthy snacks available. As you attempt to build the healthy habit of healthy snacking, always have some sort of healthy food available to nibble on should you feel the urge at home, the office, or on the go. Thinking ahead in this way will make you less likely to rationalize your way into eating something you know you shouldn't.

Of course, since you've been reading this book you've probably already begun the process of getting rid of the junk food in your kitchen. The office, however, presents a whole new battlefield of temptations. There are the free doughnuts somebody keeps bringing in each morning for anyone who's interested. Who wouldn't be interested? Those colorfully wrapped candies in bowls on your coworkers' desks also beckon for your attention. Oh, and those omnipresent vending machines. Somewhere between lunch and quitting time they begin their siren call. "Aw, c'mon," they whisper, "have a Snickers bar on me. Just one won't hurt, will it?"

Watch out for rationalizing. One today becomes one again tomorrow, and so on. We are a people who rationalize ourselves into bad habits. Prepare yourself to resist. Little habits can bring big trouble. Just one pack of Lifesavers a day will put ten pounds of unhealthy fat on your body in a year.[2]

So what kind of snacks would be good, you're asking? Here's a list of healthful snacks you might find enjoyable. As you discover more, add them to this list.

HEALTHY SNACKS

Fruit

- *Fresh*: apples, bananas, oranges, melons, peaches, pears, plums, apricots, pineapple, grapefruit, grapes
- *Dried*: apricots, figs, prunes, raisins, pineapple, banana, pear, apple, dates
- *Frozen*: fruit-juice popsicles

(Fruits are loaded with natural sugars that give a "lift" to a long day. They also are an excellent source of vitamins and minerals. If you suffer from hypoglycemia or candida, you may need to eat fewer fruits and more of the other kinds of snacks.)

Vegetable Pieces (Raw)
Carrots, celery, peppers (green, red, yellow), cucumbers, broccoli, cauliflower, tomatoes.

(Excellent source of health-promoting vitamins and minerals, especially vitamins A, C, calcium, phosphorus, potassium, and essential amino acids.)

Nuts and Seeds (Raw)
Almonds, Brazil nuts, cashews, chestnuts, filberts (hazelnuts), peanuts, pecans, pine nuts (pignolias), pistachios, pumpkin seeds, squash seeds, sunflower seeds, walnuts.

(Powerfully nutritious. Rich source of carbohydrate, protein, fiber, B vitamins, and minerals—calcium, iron, phosphorus, and potassium. Most are high in fat [70-80 percent], but it is unsaturated. Chestnuts, however, contain only 6 percent.)

Whole-Grain Cereals
Shredded Wheat, Grape Nuts, Kashi (puffed grains), oatmeal, granola.

(These are but a few that our family enjoys as snacks. These products are very tasty without sweetener, or with a few raisins. We also avoid dairy products by using a rice milk called Rice Dream. Try it, you'll like it!)

Whole-Grain Breads

Popcorn
A wonderful source of fiber. Replace butter with "Better Butter" (see "Cut Back on Dairy Products"). Try mixing one tablespoon melted butter with ½ teaspoon lemon juice. Sprinkle over popcorn and toss with brewer's yeast (in place of salt).[3]

Carob Treats

Brownies, candies, cakes.

"The American people are full of beans," writes Frances Sheridan Goulart, author of *The Carob Way to Health*. "Each year we go through 850,000 tons of cocoa beans in the form of chocolate candies, cakes, cookies, ice cream, beverages, and other chocolate confections." These products are "rich in saturated fats, sugar, caffeine, chemicals, and empty calories."[4]

An excellent substitute for chocolate, carob is made by grinding the pods of the carob tree. It contains almost three times as much calcium as milk, is low in fat, rich in protein, and high in phosphorus and potassium. Carob is also a good source of vitamins A, B_1, and B_3 and fiber. Although it is relatively sweet (46 percent natural sugar compared to 5 ½ percent for cocoa) and has a taste comparable to chocolate, it has 40 percent fewer calories than cocoa. As an added plus, carob has none of the caffeine found naturally in chocolate.[5]

Look for carob snacks sweetened with honey, maple syrup, barley malt syrup, sorghum, or rice syrup . . . and made without hydrogenated oils. Many vegetarian cookbooks contain a variety of recipes for making your own carob treats.

And Much, Much More!

Actually, this list could go on and on. There are literally *hundreds* of snacks that you can purchase or make at home that avoid the refined sugars, refined flours, and fats typical of junk-food snacks. Because this is not intended to be a cookbook, I will not attempt to list recipes. Instead, please allow me to direct your attention to the "Further Reading" list at the end of this chapter. I've listed there the names of several cookbooks that list a variety of "healthier" snacks you can make at home.

If you're looking to purchase snack foods rather than make them, the following is a partial listing of companies that tend to use healthier ingredients in their snack-food-type products. Some of these brands can be found in mainstream supermarkets. However, a health-food store is your best bet. Again, learn to read the labels!

Arrowhead Mills	Glenny's	R.J. Corr Naturals
Auburn Farms	Hain	R.W. Frookies
Barbara's Bakery	Health Valley	R.W. Knudsen
Bear Valley	Heaven Scent Natural Foods	Santa Cruz Natural
Better Way	Kettle Foods	Schiff
Bronner	Lady J	Shiloh Farms
Caroba	Lifestream Natural Foods	Snyder's of Hanover
Chico San	Little Bear Organic Foods	Sonoma
De Boles	Manna Mixins	Sovex
De Sousa	Marion Food Specialties	Spicer's International
Desert Gold	Maranatha Natural Foods	Stone Burr
Elf Liberty	Mrs. Denson's Cookie Co.	Sunfield
Erewhon	Natural Nectar	US Mills
Fearn	Nature's Warehouse	Walnut Acres
Frankly Natural	Pamela's Products	Westbrae
Garden of Eatin'	Peddler's "Offbeat Originals"	

KEY QUOTES

*Junk food. Pop food. Trash. Fun food. Call it what you will,
we'll still eat it. And if it all disappeared
from the face of the Earth tomorrow, you know what would
happen? Riots in the streets. Panic in the pantries.
Black market Twinkies! Bathtub Pepsi!
Tootsie Rolls at caviar prices! Catastrophe!*
Michael S. Lasky
The Complete Junk Food Book

*Junk food is the single largest class of pollutants
that we inflict on our bodies.*
Michael S. Lasky
The Complete Junk Food Book

*For every 100 Army inductees, there are 106 teeth
to be pulled and 600 cavities to be filled.
That's an average of one tooth and 6 cavities per man.*
Dr. Abraham Nizel
Tufts University School of Dental Medicine

*The foods that make the most popular snacks
are comforting in some way. . . . Eat "comfort foods"
that fill you up, not out.*
Dr. Lendon Smith, M.D.
Dr. Lendon Smith's Diet Plan for Teenagers

FURTHER READING

The American Vegetarian Cookbook by Marilyn Diamond (New York: Warner Books, 1990).

The Carob Way to Health (Cookbook) by Frances Sheridan Goulart (New York: Warner Books, 1982). The history, benefits, and how-to's of using carob.

The Complete Junk Food Book by Michael S. Lasky (New York: McGraw-Hill Paperbacks, 1977). A study of the health risks and psychology behind junk food, plus in-depth analysis of hundreds of junk-food products. Written with humor.

Dr. Lendon Smith's Diet Plan for Teenagers by Lendon Smith, M.D. (New York: McGraw-Hill, 1986). See chapter 4: "Snacking, Pigging Out, and Bingeing."

Out of the Sugar Rut (Cookbook) by Joanie Huggins (Phoenix, AZ: Semantodontics, Inc., 1985). See "Pies, Cakes, Cookies, Desserts," pages 328-407.

Step-by-Step to Natural Food (Cookbook) by Diane Campbell (Clearwater, FL: CC Publishers, 1979). See chapter 8: "Sweets"; chapter 9: "Desserts"; chapter 10: "Snacks."

12

CUT DOWN ON TEA AND COFFEE, EVEN DECAF

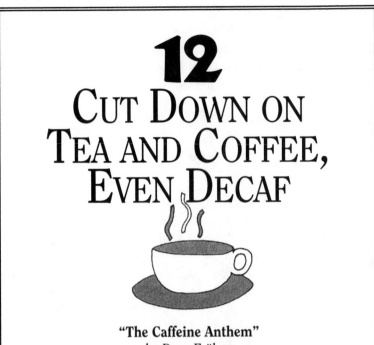

"The Caffeine Anthem"
by Dave Frähm
(sung to the tune of "The Star-Spangled Banner")

*Oh say can you see,
my cup of coffee?
It's the stuff that I need
for my fix of caffeine!
Without it I'm a mess,
my head is distressed.
My mind is all shot
'til I've had half a pot.
Oh, but now I've found it,
my headache has quit.
My brain has kicked in,
I am human again.
Oh, please don't ever try to take
caffeine away from me.
It's the drug that we crave most,
in the land of the free.*

Cars run on gas. Lights run on electricity. And Americans seem to run on coffee. Fact is, we drink more than half of the coffee produced on the planet. The Swedes drink more coffee per person than we do, but no country comes near to matching our total consumption.[1] It's there for every meal and every meeting. Committee people drink it while doing business around big tables. Business people drink it in committees that form around coffeepots during breaks. Church people drink it on Sunday mornings to stay awake in church. College students drink it on weekday nights to stay awake for studying.

Some people drink coffee for emotional comfort. Every year during tax season, H&R Block offices serve up more than 2.2 million gallons of the stuff.

For many of us, offering coffee to guests in our homes is our way of breaking the ice. Have a cup o' "joe," cup o' "java," cup o' "bean juice"? Regular or unleaded? Coffee is the oil that greases our social motors.

WHY CUT DOWN?

For whatever reasons you drink coffee, you need to do so advisably. There are certain things about coffee, and tea, for that matter, that you need to take into consideration as you think about long-term health. Those who study these things are telling us, cut down on coffee and tea, even decaffeinated.

Caffeine
Found naturally in both coffee and tea, caffeine has the potential to stimulate the onset of several health concerns.

"Coffee nerves": The caffeine in coffee is a drug, a stimulant, an "upper." Athletes are known to use it to enhance their performance, downing a few cups of coffee the morning before a big race. Its impact at the office can be anything but performance-enhancing. The caffeine consumed during that insidious custom known as "coffee break" can leave you jumpy, jittery, and nervous. It destroys vitamin B, the nerve-building vitamins, resulting in impaired concentration. Doing an "upper"

at break time, then sitting back down to resume work, just doesn't make any sense!

If consumed after the workday is over, say, following the evening meal, the caffeine in coffee has the potential to keep your mind "flying" all night, robbing you of the kind of sleep your body needs to function at top form.

Although it's referred to as "coffee nerves," consuming regular tea will have the same impact on the human nervous system—just not as quickly. A cup of tea contains about half the caffeine of a cup of coffee.

High blood pressure and irregular heartbeat: For some, this can be a dangerous condition. Donald M. Vickery, M.D., suggests that "it seems likely that these effects increase risk in someone prone to heart attack. Thus, while it seems unlikely that caffeine by itself causes heart attacks, it may be the last straw for someone on the brink of one."[2]

Elevated blood cholesterol levels: These days, we're all concerned about cholesterol and our hearts. The news from the coffeepot is not good. "I'm sorry to tell you this," writes John A. McDougall, M.D., "but coffee raises the level of cholesterol in the blood." The good news is that "people with high blood levels of cholesterol who give up this beverage show a significant drop. . . . The improvement can mean a 10% decrease, which could have a considerable impact on the danger of dying from heart disease."[3]

Vitamin and mineral depletion: Caffeine so negatively affects the vitamin and mineral reserves in the body that Stuart M. Berger, M.D., author of *Dr. Berger's Immune Power Diet*, recommends the following program of daily dietary supplementation designed to help you replace the nutrients you destroy each day you consume caffeinated beverages.

- ▶ 1000 mg. vitamin C
- ▶ 50 mg. zinc
- ▶ 400 mg. calcium
- ▶ 500 mg. magnesium
- ▶ B-complex vitamin[4]

Breast lumps: Many women are sensitive to caffeine, developing benign nodules in the breasts referred to as fibrocystic disease. There is some concern that the continual stress to breast tissue dealt by a diet high in caffeine products (coffee, tea, chocolate, cola, cocoa) might eventually cause cysts to become cancerous. Dr. McDougall points out that "some studies have indicated that women with fibrocystic disease have about three times the risk of developing breast cancer."[5]

Dr. David Steenblock, D.O., points out that a condition of sore, painful breasts in general is often due to caffeine, as well. Remove the caffeine from the diet and this painful condition disappears.

Birth defects: Caffeine has a molecular structure that allows it to cross the placenta from mother to developing child. "Caffeine has been shown to cause birth defects in animals and is suspected of causing the same defects in humans. It would follow that you should completely avoid coffee, tea, colas, and chocolate in all forms during pregnancy."[6]

Cancer
The consumption of coffee has been linked to the development of pancreatic and bladder cancers. Studies are not absolutely conclusive (few in the medical world are), but there is enough evidence linking coffee with the onset of these cancers that medical doctors conducting these studies are giving up coffee themselves. (Tea has not been implicated, suggesting that caffeine is not involved.) One such "coffee-abstaining" researcher, a Dr. Brian MacMahon, believes that his findings from a seven-year study show that as many as 20,000 cases of pancreatic cancer a year may be related to coffee drinking.[7]

Carcinogenic Chemicals
As an import from Third World countries, many coffees contain production chemicals now illegal in the United States for health reasons. In his book *Choose to Live*, author Joseph D. Weissman, M.D., points out that "coffee, along with other foods imported from Third World countries, contains significant

amounts of pesticides that are now banned in the United States, including aldrin, BHC, chlordane, DDT, and lindane."[8] It is true that there are a growing number of organically grown coffees (no pesticides) being marketed in health-food stores. Even so, you still have the caffeine and acids to deal with.

The chemicals used to remove the caffeine from coffee have also been linked with cancer. Originally, a chemical solvent called trichloroethylene, or TCE, was used for this purpose. It remained in coffee beans as part of the finished product. When it was eventually banned as a carcinogen, coffee companies switched to a new solvent—*methylene chloride*. It, too, has been linked to cancer—specifically lung and liver cancers.[9]

Oxalic Acid
Found in both regular and decaffeinated coffee, oxalic acid contributes to the potential onset of a couple of health problems.

Osteoporosis: Oxalic acid is a strong, poisonous acid that occurs in various plants. Our bodies call upon their stores of calcium to buffer and neutralize the impact of heavy acids—like oxalic acid—when they are introduced into our systems. Constant repetition of this neutralizing process robs our bones of calcium, contributing to the onset of osteoporosis—a serious weakening of the bones.

Kidney stones: The calcium released from the bones into the blood system to help neutralize the effects of acid in the digestive system eventually winds up in the kidneys. A continual flow of calcium can eventually begin to form deposits known as kidney stones.

Tannic Acid
Known also as tannin, tannic acid is found in tea and to a lesser degree in coffee. It has been linked to several potential health problems.

Poor nutrient absorption: Tannin in the system has been shown to decrease the ability of the body to absorb dietary iron.

Digestion disorders: Tannin has been known to lead to indigestion, heartburn, gastritis (inflammation of the mucous membrane of the stomach), and ulcers.

Cancer: Tannin has been linked to oral and esophageal cancer in some countries where it is consumed in large quantities.

KEY QUOTES

Even those who douse themselves with sunblock,
dabble with vegetarian diets and ditch drinking find it hard
to listen to ongoing warnings from caffeine researchers.
"Hell no," say members of the caffeine crowd,
hugging their coffee mugs and their cola cans to their
chests. It's the last bad habit. Besides, they add,
they can't function without it.
Claudia Feldman, "Hooked on Caffeine"
Your Health magazine

After the body is made toxic by a high concentration
of coffee poisons over a long period of time, coffee ceases
to stimulate, no matter how much is drunk,
and a period of depression follows.
It is a dangerous period, I believe, for the body is saturated
with poisons and very fatigued,
precisely the time when some sort of health
catastrophe may occur—arthritis, neuritis, cancer.
Henry G. Bieler, M.D.
Food Is Your Best Medicine

The casual way in which our culture uses stimulants
can easily mask the underlying problems that need your real
attention—an improper diet. If you can cut these
stimulants completely out of your life,
you'll be doing yourself a big favor.
Stuart M. Berger, M.D.
What Your Doctor Didn't Learn in Medical School

It would seem that if you're going to continue to drink tea or coffee, even decaffeinated, you ought to cut way back on the amount. At the most, drink one or two cups a day. If you're pregnant or nursing, drop these beverages altogether.

HOW TO CUT DOWN

Cutting back on coffee and tea consumption can be very, very difficult. The caffeine in these beverages is a physically addicting drug. Dr. Roland Griffiths observes what you've no doubt already experienced if you've tried at all to get off caffeine, and that is that stopping "cold turkey" "can produce a severe and clinically significant withdrawal syndrome including headache, fatigue, fuzzy thinking, mood changes and other symptoms associated with depression and anxiety."[10]

Rest as much as possible during this time, and be sure to drink lots of fluids to keep your system flushing itself out. In my own case, I slowly kept cutting back on my level of coffee consumption until I was drinking just one cup a day. At the same time I was developing an appreciation for caffeine-free herbal teas, plus water with freshly squeezed lemon. From there, the last step to zero cups of coffee was not too difficult.

In the end, no matter which approach you try you're probably going to experience some level of unpleasant withdrawal symptoms. Hang in there. These too shall pass, and you'll soon be free from one more kind of potentially health-damaging addiction.

Here are some product ideas to try as you're trying to wean yourself from caffeine.

Water-Decaffeinated Coffee
When it comes to promoting health, decaffeinated coffee is no "knight in shining armor." Although the caffeine has been dealt with, you've still got the heavy acids to protect yourself from. There's also the carcinogenic chemical solvent used in the decaffeinating process. However, in the late 1970s a company in Switzerland invented a way to remove caffeine from coffee beans using nothing but pure water. If you're trying to wean yourself from coffee and caffeine and are having a difficult time of it,

perhaps step one would be to ask for water-decaffeinated coffee at your health-food store. Once you've left caffeine behind, explore moving on to some of the following beverages.

Cereal Coffee Replacements

There are many brands sold in health-food stores these days. They don't really taste like coffee, but with a little time can become an acquired taste to replace coffee on your menu. I appreciate Dr. Dean Ornish's opinion about these products: "If you look on these as coffee *substitutes*, then you may be disappointed. If you see these as interesting beverages in their own right, then most of them taste quite good."[11]

▶ Bambu—chicory, figs, wheat, malted barley, acorns
▶ Barley Brew—100 percent barley
▶ Cafix—roasted barley, rye, chicory, and shredded beet roots
▶ Caphag—rye, oats, millet, figs, barley, chicory
▶ Dacopa—roasted syrup of the dahlia flower tuber
▶ Inka—roasted barley, rye, chicory, beet roots
▶ Kaffree Roma—roasted malt barley, roasted barley, roasted chicory
▶ Pero—roasted, ground malted barley, barley, chicory, rye, molasses
▶ Pioneer—barley, figs, chicory
▶ Postem—bran, wheat, molasses, artificial coffee flavoring
▶ Roastaroma—crystal malt, roasted barley, carob, chicory, cassia bark, star anise, allspice
▶ Sipp—roasted barley, chicory, rye, chickpea, and fig
▶ Wilson's Heritage—100 percent barley, can be brewed like coffee

Herbal Teas

Using broad categories, there are three basic kinds of teas: black, green, and herbal. Black and green are made with tea leaves and contain caffeine. Herbal is obviously made with herbs, and is therefore not really a tea but a tealike drink. Unless blended together with regular tea, it is naturally caffeine free. Read the label!

Some herbs, like those in the following list, have been linked with negative influences on the body and should not be used in herbal tea blends: borage, comfrey, coltsfoot, godolobo yerba, gravel plant, tansy ragwort, lungwort, Russian comfrey, fireweed, liferoot plant, bonesel, senecio, burdock, hydrangea, juniper, catnip, jimson weed.[12] Comfrey, coltsfoot, and sassafras in particular have been linked to cancer.[13] Again, read labels!

That said, many people do turn to safe blends of herbal teas as a naturally caffeine-free replacement to coffee or tea in their diets. They can be both calming and rejuvenating to the nervous system. Celestial Seasonings is perhaps the most popular manufacturer of herbal teas.

Hot Lemon Tonic
Drinking lots of purified water will not only help you break the caffeine habit by washing its residues out of your system, but will also help to keep your immune system strong against disease.[14] A squeeze of lemon in a cup of hot water cuts through mucus and provides a cleansing effect on your organs.

FURTHER READING

The Book of Whole Foods: Nutrition and Cuisine by Karen MacNeil (New York: Vintage Books, 1981). See "Juices, Waters, Teas, and Coffees," pages 283-300.

Choose to Live by Joseph D. Weissman, M.D. (New York: Penguin Books, 1988). See chapter 4: "Week One: Water and Beverages."

Everyday Cancer Risks and How to Avoid Them by Mary Kerney Levenstein (Garden City Park, NY: Avery Publishing Group, 1992). See chapter 4: "Caffeine."

Jane Brody's Nutrition Book by Jane Brody (New York: Bantam Books, 1981). See chapter 12: "Coffee, Tea ..."

13

CUT BACK ON SOFT DRINKS, EVEN SUGARLESS

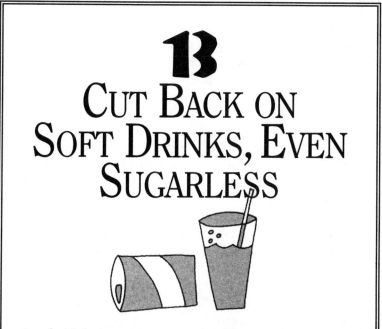

Soft drinks began appearing on the American scene back in 1849. Few took notice. The average consumption back then was less than a pint per person for the whole year.[1] Today the average American consumes over 240 pints of the stuff each year—over 30 gallons.[2] Since there are roughly 250 million of us, that means a whopping 7.5 billion gallons down the hatch.

WHY CUT BACK?

As with everything else we put into our mouths, our chief concern should be its effect upon our bodies. What we consume today determines our health tomorrow. Is soda pop a health-promoting choice? No. What about the diet kind, or the kind without sugar and caffeine? Isn't there some sort of soda pop that's okay? Not according to David Reuben, M.D., author of *Everything You Always Wanted to Know About Nutrition.* In uncompromising fashion he flatly warns, "Don't use soda pop in any form."[3]

Phosphoric Acid

The chemicals in soda pop fall under the categories of artificial flavorings, artificial color additives and dyes, acidifying agents, buffering agents, viscosity-producing agents, foaming agents, and preservatives. One of these chemical additives, *phosphoric acid*, is added to many kinds of soda pop to help keep the carbonated bubbles from going flat. Because good health depends upon our bodies being able to maintain a one-to-one balance between calcium and phosphorus in our systems, calcium is released from our teeth and bones into our bloodstreams to help balance the phosphoric acid in the pop we drink. Eventually the phosphoric acid is excreted, taking with it the released calcium. Thus, a habit of soft drink consumption actually robs our bodies of calcium, leading to a condition known as osteoporosis—soft teeth and weak bones.

Phosphoric acid is also known to neutralize the hydrochloric acid in our stomachs. This is unfortunate, for we need hydrochloric acid to help us digest our food and utilize its nutrients. It is especially required for calcium utilization.[4] So, not only does phosphoric acid leach calcium from our bones, it also prohibits hydrochloric acid from helping to restore it. Bones and teeth just can't win with this stuff in our diet.

In a survey designed to measure the amount of phosphoric acid in twenty different soft drinks, the following were found to contain the highest amounts: Tab, Coke, Diet Coke, caffeine-free Coke, and Mr. Pibb.[5] The formulas may have been changed for the better since this survey was conducted. Read labels. By the way, Pepsi Free, Diet Pepsi Free, Like Cola, 7-Up, and Mountain Dew had no phosphoric acid in them. This, however, does not mean that these products are free from the other problems true of soft drinks.

Tap Water

The main ingredient in bottled soft drinks is water, straight from the tap. We've already talked about the nasty stuff found in tap water. To the sea of chemical additives in soda pop are added things like chlorine, trihalomethanes, lead, cadmium, and organic pollutants found in abundance in our nation's water supply. Not the stuff on which good health is built.

Sugar

The sweetener in regular pop, of course, is sugar. We've already discussed the health hazards that sugar presents as part of the standard American diet (SAD). It rots teeth, impairs the immune system, and can lead to the onset of degenerative disease. If you haven't already read the "Cut Back on Refined Sugars" chapter of this book, please do so.

The manufacturers of soft drinks are the largest single user of refined sugar in this country.[6] One 12-ounce can of regular soda pop contains over an ounce of sugar (or about 7 teaspoons). "The sugar is cheap, rotten refined sugar that can only do you damage—diabetes, obesity, tooth decay, and all the rest," observes David Reuben, M.D.[7]

Aspartame

By choosing a diet soda to avoid sugar, you're consuming aspartame. Better known as NutraSweet, it is the sugar substitute used these days in diet soft drinks. Saccharin, previously used, was found to be carcinogenic, as were cyclamates before that. Many health professionals now have serious doubts as to the safety of aspartame, as well.

Andrew Weil, M.D., author of a book entitled *Natural Health, Natural Medicine,* states that "because I have seen a number of patients, mostly women, who report headaches from this substance, I don't regard it as free from toxicity. Women also find that aspartame aggravates PMS (premenstrual syndrome)."[8]

Joseph Weissman, M.D., has this warning about aspartame in diet soda: "If it is stored in warm areas or kept on store shelves for a prolonged period, aspartame will change to methanol, an alcohol that ultimately converts to formaldehyde and formic acid—known carcinogens."[9] Remember that next time you walk down the soft drink aisle in your supermarket wondering how long those cans have been sitting there, or next time you see pallets of diet soda stacked in the summer heat outside your local convenience store.

When asked which was better, regular pop or diet, Ann Donovan, a certified nutritionist, replied: "Neither! But if you were dying of thirst on a desert island and somebody offered you regular or diet with NutraSweet, go with the regular."

A local health-food store my family frequents has a policy against carrying products on their shelves that contain aspartame (NutraSweet).

Caffeine

The jitters, insomnia, high blood pressure, irregular heartbeat, elevated blood cholesterol levels, vitamin and mineral depletion, breast lumps, birth defects, perhaps some forms of cancer—these and more are part of the package deal of health problems and risks that come with choosing to consume caffeinated drinks.

Taking size into account, the impact of three cans of regular Coke a day on a seven-year-old kid is the same as an adult drinking eight cups of coffee![10] Needless to say, physicians—particularly pediatricians—are alarmed. Could it be that the consumption of caffeinated soda pop is contributing to developmental disorders, both physical and mental, in our children? There are many health professionals who would say so. One author puts it this way: "No parent would knowingly give poison to their children; and yet, every time you hand your child a soda pop or flavored drink, you are giving him chemicals that are stored in his body. Is it any wonder that twelve-year-olds die of cancer, teenagers are afflicted with MS, and young men and women commit bizarre acts?"[11]

KEY QUOTES

*In the eternal order of the universe,
man-refined sugar, like all other things,
plays its part. Perhaps the sugar pushers are our predators,
leading us into temptation, peddling a kind of sweet,
sweet, human pesticide which lures greedy seekers*

into self-destruction, weeding the human garden,
naturally selecting the fittest for survival while the rest go
down in another biblical flood—not water this time,
but Coke, Pepsi, and Dr. Pepper—
purifying the human race for a new age.
William Duffy
Sugar Blues

The Soft Drink Association boasts that 85%
of the hospitals they surveyed serve soft drinks routinely
to the patients. Is it any wonder that we can't get well?
Diane Campbell
Step-by-Step to Natural Food

You can drink Coke every day all day long
and not get tired of it. 15 minutes after you've finished
a Coke, you're a new customer again,
and that's where we get you.
E. J. Kahn
The Big Drink

The National Soft Drink Association promotes
sugary soda pop to children in literature that claims
soda is a good source of water.
In that case, it would be better to drink the water.
Michael Jacobson, Ph.D.
Executive Director of the Center for Science
in the Public Interest

HOW TO CUT BACK

It would seem that the bottom line here is to stay away from soda pop. At least cut way back. Neither regular nor diet does your body any good. In fact, a steady habit of soda consumption can do a great deal of harm. You ought to be making every effort to wean yourself from it completely. How to do it, though—that's the problem. Here are two tips.

Freshly Made Juices
Consider purchasing a juicer and making your own fresh juices at home from fresh, organic fruits and vegetables. We use a Champion juicer ourselves, well known for its ability to masticate out every drop of juice from the produce. It's "tops" with many nutritionists, although there are other excellent brands on the market.

The important enzymes in fresh juice begin to die soon after they're exposed to oxygen. In order to get the most health benefit, either drink the juice soon after preparation or put it in a tightly sealed thermos for later. Anne and I credit the incredible health effects of juicing as a key element in a cancer-fighting strategy that helped her beat terminal cancer. For more details see our book *A Cancer Battle Plan*, published by Piñon Press.

Soft Drinks with All the Right Stuff
Or rather, without all the bad stuff. You'll want a product made from purified water and fresh fruit juices, plus free from artificial sweeteners, refined sugar, artificial colorings and flavorings, preservatives, and caffeine. The fewer the chemical additives, the better.

Try making your own soda pop. Mix club soda or sparkling mineral water with various combinations of freshly squeezed fruit juice.

FURTHER READING

Choose to Live by Joseph D. Weissman, M.D. (New York: Penguin Books, 1988). See chapter 4: "Week One: Water and Beverages."

Everything You Always Wanted to Know About Nutrition by David Reuben, M.D. (New York: Simon and Schuster, 1978). See pages 254, 255.

Step-by-Step to Natural Food by Diane Campbell (Clearwater, FL: CC Publishers, 1979). See Chapter 11: "Beverages."

14
CUT DOWN ON ALCOHOL

Surveys indicate that well over one-third of all Americans, 90 million or so, are considered "social drinkers."[1] This is generally defined as liking alcohol and having a habit of using it on a moderate basis. Another 10 million are considered alcoholics. They've gone beyond just an enjoyable habit to physical and psychological addiction.

If you're one who uses alcohol and are truly concerned about developing healthy habits, you need to take a long, hard look at whether or not alcohol consumption is worth it. First of all, its collective effect upon our society is devastating. Estimates are that alcohol is responsible for nearly $45 billion a year in industrial losses—sickness, poor decision making, accidents, etc. It is also an active agent in 50 percent of all traffic deaths, 30 percent of small-aircraft accidents, and 66 percent of all violent crimes.[2] Many consider alcohol the most dangerous and devastating of legally gotten drugs in our nation.

Secondly, and perhaps more importantly, you need to consider its impact upon your body. The question that is usually asked concerning alcohol is, "How much is too much?" Too much for what? If the question concerns nutrition, alcohol not only gives nothing to our bodies, it takes away. It's "worse than useless," write Allan Luks and Joseph Barbato in their book *You Are What You Drink*. "It not only fails to add to daily nutritional requirements, but actually interferes with good eating habits and with the body's ability to use the nutrients in the other foods that we consume."[3]

WHY CUT DOWN?

Can a person get away with a drink now and then without it doing much harm? Perhaps. But what exactly what does "now and then" mean? Are we talking a drink or two a week, or a two to three every night after work? Here's just a partial list of the many health negatives associated with excessive consumption of alcoholic beverages.

Depressed Immune System Function
Research now clearly shows that excessive amounts of alcohol in the bloodstream result in loss of white blood cells, which fight off foreign invaders and cancerous cells.[4]

Depressed Heart Function
Alcohol reduces your heart's working capacity. According to Nathan Pritikin, a well-known health educator and researcher, "just two cocktails will cut it by about 20% for about 24 hours. If you're a two-drink-a-day person, you've already deprived yourself of ⅕ of your heart."[5]

Allergic Reactions
According to the Center of Science in the Public Interest, as many as 20 million of us may be allergic to the other ingredients besides alcohol in wine, beer, and distilled spirits.[6] "It is astonishing how many people find that alcoholic beverages not only go to their heads but also to their skin and gastrointestinal and respiratory systems," observes allergist Claude A. Frazer, M.D., author of *Coping with Food Allergy*.[7]

Vitamin and Mineral Deficiency
Alcohol uses up nutrients, leaving our stores depleted. It robs our bodies of vitamins C and A, folic acid and other B vitamins, potassium, magnesium, iron, and zinc.[8]

Cancer
The excessive consumption of alcoholic beverages has been linked to the development of a variety of cancers, including those of the throat, mouth, larynx, pharynx, esophagus, bladder, breast, pancreas, head, neck, and liver.

In addition, Patrick Quillin, Ph.D., R.D., reports in his book *Healing Nutrients* that "in a study of over 8,000 men ... those who consumed more than 16 ounces of beer daily had an increased risk of rectal cancer. Wine and whisky consumption were related to an increased risk of lung cancer."[9]

Many alcoholic beverages have also been found to contain pesticide residues from sprayed fruits or grains, plus another cancer-causing agent called urethane which forms in alcoholic drinks as the result of naturally occurring chemical reactions. It has been found in American bourbon whiskeys, European fruit brandies, cream sherries, port, sake, and Chinese wines.[10]

Stroke
In the study reported above by Patrick Quillin, drinkers had more than twice the rate of strokes as nondrinkers. Heavy drinkers experienced five times more strokes than nondrinkers.[11]

Hypertension (High Blood Pressure)
Of course, part of the reason for strokes is a rupture in a blood vessel in the brain. This is often the result of high blood pressure. Excessive consumption of alcoholic beverages raises blood pressure.[12]

Osteoporosis
When alcoholic beverages are consumed, calcium is drained from our bones and teeth in order to help alkalinize their acid. Studies show that alcohol consumption also actually interferes

with calcium absorption from other foods. Social drinkers are two and a half times more likely to develop osteoporosis than nondrinkers. People who consume alcohol in excess are sure to develop the disease.[13]

Liver Problems

In her book *The Nutrition Detective*, Nan Kathryn Fuchs, Ph.D., points out that "alcohol makes it more difficult for the liver to work properly. And, if your liver isn't working properly, it is more difficult to produce the enzyme that metabolizes alcohol in the liver." You wind up caught in a vicious circle. She goes on to say that "a healthy liver can handle only 2 to 3 teaspoons of alcohol an hour . . . (taking) as long as 24 hours to eliminate the alcohol and the by-products from just one drink."[14]

Excessive alcohol consumption can eventually lead to cirrhosis of the liver, the seventh-leading cause of death in the United States.[15] Men who consume three drinks a day, and women who drink only half that much, are at increased risk for developing this disease.[16] Cirrhosis is a scarring of the liver in which normal cells are damaged and replaced by scar tissue, which keeps the liver from carrying on its vital functions properly. It is an irreversible condition, often making its presence known only when things have reached crisis proportions.

Birth Defects

The surgeon general of the United States has been warning women since the early 1980s to abstain from all alcohol use while pregnant. Heavy drinking while pregnant can lead to FAS, fetal alcohol syndrome. This involves permanent physical and mental damage to the fetus, worst cases resembling Down's syndrome. According to Dr. David Steenblock, D.O., even men who consume alcohol run the risk of producing children with FAS.

Even at very low levels of consumption (0.1 ounce a day), alcohol can have negative neurological results on unborn children.[17]

Alcohol has the potential to damage every system in our

bodies by destroying or depressing the proper functioning of the cells and organs that comprise them. In her book *Everyday Cancer Risks and How to Avoid Them,* author Mary Kerney Levenstein points out that alcohol has been linked to damage of the central nervous system, the gastrointestinal system, the circulatory system, the musculoskeletal system, the reproductive system, and the immune system.[18]

Bottom line, drinking alcoholic beverages is just not a healthy habit.

KEY QUOTES

If you have an occasional drink you may be getting away without doing yourself much harm. If you're a steady drinker and think you're healthy, you're fooling yourself.
Nan Kathryn Fuchs, Ph.D.
The Nutrition Detective

Any potential beneficial effects of alcohol are far outweighed by its harmful ones.
Joseph D. Weissman, M.D.
Choose to Live

Alcohol is the strongest and most toxic of the common psychoactive substances. It is a "hard" drug, harder than heroin, cocaine, LSD, and all the other illegal drugs. Our culture promotes and encourages the use of alcohol and gives the false impression that it is not as dangerous as the disapproved drugs.
Andrew Weil, M.D.
Natural Health, Natural Medicine

Excess alcohol will eventually kill most people in a variety of ways.
Patrick Quillin Ph.D., R.D.
Healing Nutrients

HOW TO CUT DOWN

Here are some ideas that will help you cut down or cut out altogether your consumption of alcohol.

1. *Give your body alcohol-free days.* If you're an everyday drinker, begin to cut back by giving yourself at least two to three alcohol-free days a week.

2. *Learn other ways to relax.* Many people turn to alcoholic beverages to help them relax from the emotional stress of life. Ironically, excessive drinking reduces the body's absorption of certain B vitamins that help our nervous systems deal effectively with stress. It is important, therefore, to learn other ways than alcohol for handling life's tensions.

Exercise is the most beneficial. Not only does it release certain morphinelike chemicals from your brain called endorphins that give you a sense of well-being, but it also helps to strengthen your entire physical system. Some refer to exercise as "brewing your own high" without the help of alcohol.

3. *Switch to nonalcoholic "taste-alikes."* There are a growing number of beverages on the market that taste like beer, wine, and so on, but don't have alcohol in them.

4. *Seek professional help.* Contact an alcoholism support group and/or treatment center for help. Check in the yellow pages in your phone book under "Alcoholism Information and Treatment." Robert Gleser, M.D., author of *The HealthMark Program for Life*, suggests that if you drink every day, ask yourself why. You may have a problem. The greatest danger with alcohol is denial.

KEY QUESTION

Q. I've heard that drinking a little alcohol each day is good for you. Any truth to that?

A. Joseph D. Weissman, M.D.: "Doctors disagree about the value of alcohol consumed in limited amounts. Some reports indicate that alcohol in small amounts raises levels of high density lipoproteins (HDL) (considered the good kind of cholesterol), which are presumed to protect against artery disease. However, it raises levels of HDL3, a subgroup of high density lipoproteins that do not offer this protection. It is HDL2 that decreases the risk of coronary disease."[19]

Robert A. Gleser, M.D.: "The only ways you can realistically raise your HDL's are to exercise, lose weight, and stop smoking."[20]

FURTHER READING

Cancer and Nutrition by Charles B. Simone, M.D. (New York: McGraw-Hill, 1983). See chapter 10: "Alcohol and Caffeine."

Choose to Live by Joseph D. Weissman, M.D. (New York: Penguin Books, 1988). See "Alcohol," pages 34-35.

Everyday Cancer Risks and How to Avoid Them by Mary Kerney Levenstein (Garden City Park, NY: Avery Publishing Group, 1992). See chapter 3: "Alcohol."

Jane Brody's Nutrition Book by Jane Brody (New York: Bantam Books, 1981). See chapter 14: "Alcohol: Nutrient or Nemesis?"

Natural Health, Natural Medicine by Andrew Weil, M.D. (Boston: Houghton Mifflin, 1990). See "Addiction to Legal Drugs," pages 133-135.

You Are What You Drink by Allan Luks and Joseph Barbato (New York: The Stonesong Press, 1989).

15
QUIT SMOKING

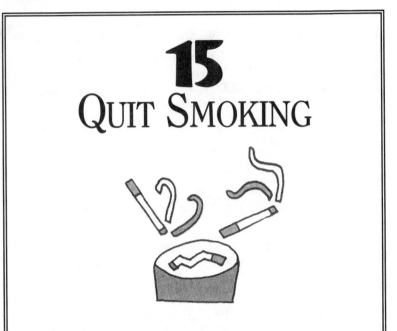

I n the United States today, 50 million smokers annually light up approximately 600 billion cigarettes, 4 billion cigars, and 11 billion pipefuls of tobacco.[1] Studies show that over 85 percent of those who smoke want to quit.[2] It's not impossible. In fact, over 40 million Americans have already done so.[3] If you smoke, you need to seriously consider joining the ranks of those who have kicked the habit.

WHY QUIT?

The reason you should quit, of course, is because smoking is clearly related to several nasty diseases. An explanation of the link between these diseases and smoking follows.

Cancer
There are over 36,000 chemicals formed in the 950 degree Fahrenheit heat at the tip of a cigarette.[4] Tobacco smoke contains stuff like benzopyrenes, formaldehyde, nitrosamines, hydrogen cyanide, aromatic hydrocarbons, phenols, and polo-

nium 210 (a radioactive element)—all poisons, many of them carcinogenic.[5] The label on the side of cigarette packs tells it all: "Warning: Smoking *causes* cancer."

The primary cancer associated with smoking tobacco is lung cancer. It is the number-one killer among cancers today. Two packs a day will increase your chances fifteen to twenty-five times of developing lung cancer. Studies show that one pack a day is likely to cut your life short by seven years. One out of every three smokers will die as many as twenty-one years before his or her time.[6]

Smoking tobacco in all forms (cigarettes, cigars, pipe) is also linked to cancers of the lip, tongue, salivary glands, larynx, pharynx, esophagus, mouth, bladder, kidney, colon, rectum, pancreas, and cervix. Chewing tobacco is a major cause of cancer of the cheek and gum.

Lung cancer has become the leading killer of American women. It claims more lives each year than dreaded breast cancer.[7] Most of it, according to the American Cancer Society, is attributed to smoking. In the 1980s a popular cigarette aimed at the female market proclaimed, "You've come a long way, baby." Perhaps "You've come the wrong way" is more appropriate!

According to the World Health Organization, smoking causes nearly 400,000 deaths (males included) each year in the United States. That's nearly 1,100 a day—46 every hour. More people die every year because of tobacco smoke than the total number of Americans killed in World War I, World War II, and the Vietnam War combined![8]

Heart Disease
Smoking is right up there with high blood pressure and elevated levels of blood cholesterol as a risk factor in heart attacks. The nicotine in tobacco smoke stimulates our adrenal glands to produce adrenaline. It reaches the heart, causing it to work harder and thus demand increased oxygen. Unfortunately, tobacco smoke also contains carbon monoxide. It bonds with the red blood cells that normally carry oxygen to the heart,

pushing the oxygen out. The overworked, underoxygenated heart finds itself under extreme stress.

Chronic Obstructive Lung Disease

In their book *The Well Adult*, Mike Samuels, M.D., and wife Nancy describe this third major area of illness caused by smoking. They point out that most people who smoke have "significant changes" in their airways and lungs. "Smoking paralyzes the cilia, the microscopic fingerlike projections that move particles and debris out of the lungs and throat. Moreover, smokers' lungs are chronically inflamed and contain unusually high numbers of white blood cells, whose function is to break down foreign particles and dead cells. Ultimately these white blood cells even break down cells in the lung itself, causing lung tissue to be less elastic, which in turn makes breathing more difficult."[9]

"Smoker's cough" is the result of this long-term lung inflammation turning into chronic bronchitis.

Chronic Fatigue

Besides the risks of eventually developing cancer, heart disease, and chronic lung disorders, smoking drains the body of energy for daily living. Not only is our heart overburdened with the double whammy of nicotine and carbon monoxide described above, but so is every cell in our bodies. Our entire system is being asked to work harder, yet with less oxygen to fuel itself. Cells need oxygen to convert nutrients into energy. Without it, they become sluggish and eventually die. Holly Atkinson, M.D., author of *Women and Fatigue*, points out that "every time you take a puff you are asphyxiating yourself. It is no wonder fatigue is one of the major effects of cigarette smoking."[10]

Secondhand (Passive) Smoke

If you don't quit smoking for yourself, do it for those around you whom you care about. Here are some facts that may influence your decision:

▸ In 1986 the U.S. surgeon general, C. Everett Koop, authored a report entitled *The Health Consequences of Involuntary Smoking*. In it, passive (sidestream) smoke was characterized as even more hazardous than primary (mainstream) smoke.[11]

▸ Sidestream smoke has been shown to contain twice the tar, twice the nicotine, and five times as much carbon monoxide as mainstream smoke. Plus a new study says that people sitting in a room filled with cigarette smoke retain the dangerous chemicals (end product of nicotine) they inhale more than twice as long as the people doing the smoking.[12]

▸ A 1990 EPA report concluded that 53,000 nonsmokers are killed every year due to the effects of passive smoke.[13]

▸ A study reported in 1992 found a 30 percent increase in cancer risk among nonsmokers who lived, worked, and socialized with smokers.[14] In fact, wives of men who smoke live an average of four years less than wives of men who don't.[15]

▸ Children of smoking parents are much more likely to develop respiratory illnesses such as bronchitis, pneumonia, and asthma than those of nonsmoking parents.[16]

▸ Children born to women who smoked during pregnancy are characterized by smaller birth weight, higher incidence of infant death, more birthing complications, and infant addiction to nicotine. Added to this, a 1991 study revealed that children born to smoking mothers "scored significantly lower on academic tests as well as tests on perception, language, speech, and motor skills."[17]

Other Related Maladies
Besides robbing your body of vitamin C, smoking is linked to increased sudden death from heart arrhythmias (spasms), aortic aneurysms (weaknesses in the wall of the aorta), and blood vessel problems of the arms and legs (peripheral vascular disease). It is also associated with toxic metal poisoning of the liver (arsenic, cadmium, nickel).

KEY QUOTES

Cigarette smoking is the largest preventable public health problem currently existing in the United States.
Committee on Cigarette Smoking
and Cardiovascular Disease

If you do not smoke, don't start; if you do smoke, you should do anything possible to stop.
Joseph D. Weissman, M.D.
Choose to Live

Some people do get away with it, but smoking is a crapshoot with the dice heavily loaded against you.
Isadore Rosenfeld, M.D.
Modern Prevention, The New Medicine

There are few habits as deadly as the morning cups of coffee accompanied by several cigarettes.
Harold W. Harper, M.D., and Michael L. Culbert
How You Can Beat the Killer Diseases

Smoking-related diseases are such important causes of disability and premature death in developed countries that the control of cigarette smoking could do more to improve health and prolong life in these countries than any other single action in the whole field of preventative medicine.
World Health Organization

HOW TO QUIT

Smoking is addictive, both physically and emotionally. Most of the 40 million or so people who have successfully quit at the time of this writing have done so with great difficulty. No matter how much you want to let go of it, the habit doesn't usually want to let go of you without a tremendous fight. Perhaps you are already aware of this fact. Perhaps you've tried and failed before. If so, let me encourage you. The fact that you've already tried shows that you've taken the first huge step forward on your journey—you've responded with positive action to the truth about smoking. So what if you've regressed? Quitting is a process, a journey toward better health. No change in life is easy, but if it's truly worth making, then it's worth picking yourself up again and again till you reach your goal. Don't quit trying to quit until you've quit!

There is no right or best way to go about successfully beating the tobacco habit. But for all those who genuinely wish to make a go of it, here are a few pointers that may help you toward your goal.

Be Mentally Prepared for What You'll Face

Kicking the tobacco habit is like going to war. To be effective you will need to know what sort of things you'll be facing on the battlefield. When you quit smoking, your body will go through a period of detoxification in which the withdrawal from nicotine and other poisons may leave you with any number of very unenjoyable symptoms. These may include headaches, nausea, fatigue, nervousness, sinus congestion, panic attacks, and seemingly uncontrollable desires to binge on certain foods. It's important to remember that these things can and do eventually pass. And although you may feel like you're getting sicker, your body is actually getting healthier as the toxic build-up in your cells is released into your bloodstream for removal.

Besides these physical battles, there will also be the emotional and psychological struggles. For most smokers, smoking becomes a way to deal with the stresses of life—a comfort mechanism. If this is true of you, you'll be faced with the need to find new ways of handling stress effectively.

Make a Battle Plan that Suits You

Some people prefer to battle alone. Others find it easier to make changes within the context of a support group. Studies show that women tend to be most successful at winning their war on smoking when they're in a group situation, particularly when it's an all-female group.[18] Do what works for you. Support groups can be found by calling your local branch of the American Cancer Society or the American Heart Association.

Mary Kerney Levenstein also lists the following smoke-quitting organizations in her book *Everyday Cancer Risks and How to Avoid Them*.[19] These organizations promote certain smoke-quitting programs that have met with some success. Write or call for more information. With a little investigation you might find just the program that will help you kick the habit.

Damon and Grace Corporation
P.O. Box 674
Okemos, MI 48805-0674
(800)4-Habits

American Cancer Society
1599 Clifton Road NE
Atlanta, GA 30329
(404)320-3333

SmokeEnders
37 North 3rd Street
Easton, PA 18047
(215)250-0700

American Health Foundation
1 Dana Road
Valhalla, NY 10595
(914)592-2600

Make a Commitment to Winning the War
At this point you've carefully thought through what you're about to face. You've also come up with a plan that you think (hope) will work. Now it's time to make a commitment to winning. Set a firm date and begin your war.

Dr. Holly Atkinson tells the story of her own war to quit smoking. "The most important step in quitting," she contends, "is to make a commitment. It does not matter how long it takes you to stop, as long as you are in the process of trying."[20]

Don't Worry About Losing a Battle
In other words, if you slip up and smoke a few, pick yourself up and get back into the war. You're not defeated, just detoured. You've been making progress in the war. All is not lost. Give yourself credit for the number of hours, days, weeks, or months

that you've gone already without smoking. You won't win every battle, but you can still win the war. Forgive yourself, get yourself back on track, and quit smoking again.

Keep Reminding Yourself of the Spoils of Victory
You're not just trying to kill off a dirty, expensive, health-destroying habit, you're also trying to win back some very important territory for your health. The minute you quit smoking your body begins to repair the damage done to your lungs and other body tissues. Correspondingly, your risk for cancer and heart disease begins to go down. As new levels of oxygen are transported throughout your body, your cells and various organs will be rejuvenated. Eventually you will experience a new energy for life, along with a sense of personal pride at overcoming a very destructive habit.

Keep Doing the Little Things that Make for Victory

- Make a list of the reasons you want to quit, and refer to it often.
- Write down arguments the "addict" in you might use to convince you to smoke (e.g., "You'll never feel relaxed and comfortable as a nonsmoker—might as well enjoy your addiction"). Write rebuttals to these arguments and refer to them when you're struggling (e.g., "It's just a matter of time—maybe only several days—until you'll feel comfortable and grateful as a nonsmoker").
- Rid your house, car, and office desk of tobacco products.
- Begin a regular exercise program.
- Keep busy with various hands-on projects.
- Increase activities where you can't smoke, such as exercising, going to the movies, etc.
- Call a friend who will help talk you out of temptation.
- Reach for gum or low-calorie foods.
- Drink lots of fluids.
- Temporarily avoid places where you know others will be smoking.

- ▶ Keep track of your number of smokeless days, weeks, etc., and reward yourself (not with a cigarette) for your efforts.
- ▶ Never think you can smoke just one cigarette; you're almost certain to start smoking again.

FURTHER READING

Choose to Live by Joseph D. Weissman, M.D. (New York: Penguin Books, 1988). See "Tobacco," pages 30-34.

Everyday Cancer Risks and How to Avoid Them by Mary Kerney Levenstein (Garden City Park, NY: Avery Publishing Group, 1992). See chapter 33: "Smoking: Active and Passive."

The Heart Book by researchers at the Duke University Medical Center, Coordinator: Siegfried Heyden, M.D. (New York: Delair Publishing Co., 1981). Contains several valuable chapters.

The Well Adult by Mike Samuels, M.D., and Nancy Samuels (New York: Summit Books, 1988). See "Smoking and Health," pages 134-147.

You Can Stop by Jacquelyn Rogers (New York: Pocket Books, 1977). Written by ex-smoker, cofounder of SmokeEnders, helps you to see that you can quit.

16
EXERCISE REGULARLY

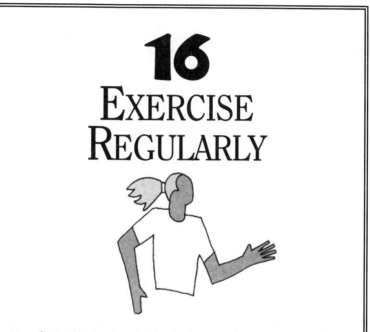

S o far in this book we've looked primarily at nutrition, things we put into our mouths. And rightly so. For what we feed our bodies is of supreme importance to our health. But as important as good nutrition is, it can only take us so far without exercise. They're inseparable partners as far as our long-term well-being is concerned.

The human body was made for action. It is perhaps the one machine in all the world that works better and gets stronger the more we use it. Muscles were made for movement. Without exercise we begin to slowly deteriorate. Like a car parked in the driveway and never used, rest brings rust. The "couch potato" syndrome that so many of us fall into leads not only to *physical* decline, but *mental* and *emotional* decay as well.

WHY EXERCISE?

If your life is worth living—if you've got things to do, places to go, and people to see before it's all over—then you need to make exercise a regular part of your routine. Here are some specific benefits a regular exercise program offers.

Improves Circulation
Exercise strengthens our heart muscle and gets our blood moving more efficiently throughout our bodies. The better our circulation, the more effectively nutrients are delivered to every one of our trillions of cells. Good health begins at the cellular level.

Improves Metabolism
Metabolism is the rate at which our cells burn up calories for energy. Exercise stimulates digestion and improves metabolism. In fact, studies indicate that a person who exercises regularly can increase his or her body's metabolic rate by 30 percent.[1]

Guards Against Weight Gain
Improved metabolism helps to control weight. In fact, all truly effective weight-loss programs involve an exercise program within their framework.

Guards Against Heart Attacks and Strokes
Studies show that regular exercise raises the level of HDL cholesterol produced in the body (the good kind), which in turn helps to lower the level of LDL cholesterol (the bad kind that clogs arteries and leads to heart attacks and strokes).[2]

Exercising also helps to lower blood pressure. Not only does it do this by dilating our arteries, but it also causes the release of endorphins from our pituitary gland. These are morphine-like hormones that lower our blood pressure and promote a state of relaxation.

In terms of guarding against heart attack, exercise also helps to strengthen the function of the heart muscle itself.

Guards Against Cancer
Regular exercise helps to keep the immune system strong, our primary defense against cancer cells. It also helps to speed up

metabolism and the elimination of wastes, thus helping to prevent colon and rectal cancers.

The increased oxygenation of our cells is yet another way in which exercise helps to guard against cancer. Dr. Otto Warburg, two-time Nobel Prize winner for his work with cells, discovered that cancerous cells are anaerobic, meaning that they thrive on fermentation as opposed to oxygen. Cancerous cells cannot thrive in an oxygenated environment.[3]

Finally, exercise helps to lower the levels of the female hormone estrogen, a high level of which is linked to the development of breast cancer.

Guards Against Osteoporosis

In his book *The HealthMark Program for Life*, Robert A. Gleser, M.D., writes that "exercise, especially weight-bearing exercise, makes strong bones by retaining calcium in the bones, thus preventing osteoporosis."[4]

Neutralizes the Effects of Stress

As already mentioned, exercise stimulates the pituitary gland at the base of the brain to release hormones called endorphins into our bloodstream. These have a tranquilizing effect upon our bodies and are released after about thirty minutes of aerobic exercise (explained below). The sense of being emotionally "up" although perhaps physically drained from a workout has given rise to the term "runners' high." Exercise plays a significant role in helping your body change its response to emotional stress.

Exercise also gives one a sense of personal accomplishment. Many agree that a little discipline in this area of life spills over into other areas, boosting one's self-image.

Other Benefits

Increased lung capacity, lower breathing rate, lower heart rate at rest, lower heart rate during exercise, lower triglyceride levels, lower uric acid levels, decreased platelet stickiness, increased muscle strength, increased flexibility, increased skill, increased muscle capacity, increased insulin-receptor sensitivity, increased energy and enthusiasm for life, improved functioning of all organs, improved elimination via skin-lungs-bowels, improved coordination.

KEY QUOTES

With regular physical activity,
a person can reduce six of eleven coronary risk factors
listed by the American Heart Association.
Ken Cooper, M.D.
The Aerobics Program for Total Well-Being

The heart is a muscle, and just like any other muscle,
if you don't use it, you lose it.
Harvey Diamond
Fit for Life

The problem is one of priorities.
Exercise must have top priority,
one that supersedes
everything except your spouse, your children,
and the food you eat. The excuse
of not being able to find the time is a cop-out.
We find time to sleep because it is mandatory.
So is exercise.
Nathan Pritikin
The Pritikin Program for Diet and Exercise

You don't have to suffer to feel good. You can make exercise
a "playout" instead of a workout.
I play tennis whenever I can because I enjoy the game
and I like the way it makes me feel afterwards.
And I walk daily. I have more energy and endurance
when I exercise regularly.
Dean Ornish, M.D.
Dr. Dean Ornish's Program for Reversing Heart Diseases

HOW TO EXERCISE REGULARLY

So how does a person go about the lifestyle change of making exercise a regular part of his or her life?

See What Condition Your Condition Is In

Many health professionals recommend that if you've been leading a rather sedentary lifestyle, you ought to get a physical exam before starting any sort of rigorous exercise program. Dr. Charles B. Simone warns: "Because of a risk of sudden death associated with beginning to exercise, anyone 35 or older, or under 35 with cardiac risk factors, should be medically screened."[5]

Dr. Joseph Weissman advocates that no matter what your age, if your cholesterol level is 200 or above, you need to be very cautious as you begin to exercise.[6]

Choose an Aerobic Exercise or Exercises that You Enjoy

According to the dictionary, the word *aerobic* means "living, active, or occurring only in the presence of oxygen." Aerobic exercise is designed to increase oxygen intake in order to stimulate and strengthen heart and lung activity. It involves large muscle groups, needs to be maintained continuously over a period of time, and is rhythmical in nature.[7] Examples include aerobic dancing, cycling (both on the road and stationary), brisk walking, cross-country skiing, hiking, jogging, jumping rope, rowing, running, skating, swimming, and "rebounding" (trampolining). There are also many health clubs that set up circuits of weight-lifting machines that offer an excellent aerobic workout, if you don't stop to rest in between machines.

Important note: The *least* beneficial of the above types of aerobic exercises are those that can potentially cause damage to muscles or joints. Jogging or running fits this description. Great for the heart, potentially bad for the knees.

Develop a Routine

Frequency: Many health-care professionals advocate vigorous exercise three to seven days a week. Most agree that three days a week is the very least you can do and still hope to remain healthy over an extended period of time. Dr. Gleser notes that "3 days is the barest minimum and is a maintenance level rather than a level used to achieve fitness."[8] Obviously, to increase your physical fitness (being and looking "in shape") you will want to increase the number of exercise days in your weekly schedule. Dr. Gordon Tessler recommends exercising at least six days a week.[9]

Intensity: A simple rule employed by all health professionals is to subtract your age from 220 to get your "maximum heart rate" (MHR). For instance, if you're forty, your MHR would be 180 beats per minute. Your "target heart rate" (THR) to shoot for while working out is between 60 and 85 percent of your MHR, or in this case between 108 and 144 beats per minute.

▸ Example: forty-year-old
▸ Average shape—Exercise at 60 percent of MHR or 108 beats per minute
▸ Good shape—Exercise at 70 percent of MHR or 126 beats per minute
▸ Excellent shape—Exercise at 85 percent of MHR or 153 beats per minute

For the first several weeks, or even months, of your exercise program you will want to keep your workouts on the low side of your target heart rate. Every fifteen minutes or so, check your pulse for six seconds and add a zero. If you're below your THR, exert yourself more. If you're above and are experiencing dizziness, slow down a bit. As your body becomes stronger, increase your pulse rate toward the high side of your THR.

Duration: In his book *Dr. Dean Ornish's Program for Reversing Heart Disease*, Dr. Ornish suggests that for "an optimal training effect, exercise continuously for 30-60 minutes at your target heart rate, not including warm-up or cool-down periods."[10] He also recommends that the priority is to increase duration before increasing intensity. In other words, if you have to exert yourself a little less in order to exercise for longer periods, do so. The ultimate goal, according to many health professionals, is to reach a point of physical conditioning at which you can exercise safely for an hour at the upper end of your target heart rate.

KEY QUESTION

Q. Since exercising increases the amount of good cholesterol in my body, which helps to clean out the bad, won't I be able to get away with continuing to eat a high-fat, high-cholesterol diet?

A. "That's precisely what Jim Fixx thought," write Dale and Kathy Martin in their book *Living Well*. "He was the author of *The Complete Book of Running*, and one of the gurus of running back in the 1970's. He ran an average of some 10 miles a day and looked like a greyhound, yet he dropped dead in his early 50's from heart disease caused by atherosclerosis."[11]

At the point in his life when Jim became concerned about exercise, he should've been equally concerned about his diet, but he wasn't. He continued to eat high-fat, high-cholesterol foods. In spite of his physical prowess, his diet was his undoing.

A similar story is told by Dr. Dean Ornish. He tells of being an intern in the emergency room at Massachusetts General Hospital in Boston the day that a thirty-seven-year-old man with a very athletic physique was wheeled in unconscious and in the midst of a massive heart attack.

Then I noticed he was wearing a World Series ring. Someone else recognized that he was Tony Conigliaro, formerly a star baseball player with the Boston Red Sox. Because his heart had stopped for at least 5 minutes before he arrived in the emergency room, he remained in a coma for the next 3 weeks. Unfortunately, he never fully recovered. He was a tragic example that a person can be very fit,

muscular, even a world-class athlete, and yet still
have a lot of blockages in his coronary arteries."[12]

I started off this chapter by saying that good nutrition without
exercise can only get you so far down the road toward excellent
health. We've now come full circle. Exercise without good nutrition is equally inadequate for excellent health and well-being.

Exercise is an extremely important part of overall health.
Without it our bodies begin to deteriorate prematurely. At the
same time, it must be accompanied by a switch to a low-fat,
low-cholesterol diet if long-term health is to be experienced.

FURTHER READING

Cancer and Nutrition by Charles B. Simone, M.D. (New
    York: McGraw-Hill, 1983). See chapter 14: "Exercise and
    Relaxation."
Dr. Dean Ornish's Program for Reversing Heart Disease
    by Dean Ornish, M.D. (New York: Ballantine Books,
    1990). See chapter 12: "How to Exercise."
The HealthMark Program for Life by Robert A. Gleser,
    M.D. (New York: McGraw-Hill, 1988). See chapter 6:
    "Getting the Most out of Exercise."
The Lazy Person's Guide to Better Nutrition by Gordon S.
    Tessler, Ph.D. (San Diego, CA: Better Health Publishers,
    1984). See chapter 11: "Exercise: Use It or Lose It."
The Well Adult by Mike Samuels, M.D., and Nancy Samuels
    (New York: Summit Books, 1988). See chapter 6:
    "Exercise and Health."

17
GET SOME SUN REGULARLY, BUT CAREFULLY

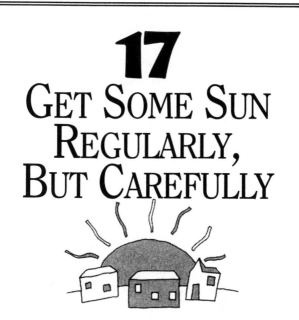

The sun that God has hung in our sky to warm our planet, clean our water through evaporation, and make plant life grow is at the same time a very important nutrient for our bodies. In fact, many consider the sun our very best source of vitamin D, a substance vital to the absorption and use of calcium.[1] If calcium is not being effectively absorbed and utilized because of a lack of vitamin D, the results can range all the way from muscle spasms and irritability to advanced bone mass loss in adults (osteoporosis), rickets in children (stunted bone growth, bowed legs, malformed teeth, protruding abdomen), and colon and rectal cancers. Calcium joins with fats in our colon and helps transfer them out of our bodies.[2]

You and I have been designed by our Creator with a fluid called ergosterol found just below our skin. When ultraviolet rays of the sun come into contact with this substance, it is converted into vitamin D and absorbed directly into our bloodstream.[3] What an ingenious way to ensure vitamin D availability and the utilization of calcium!

Today's fortified dairy products are another source of vitamin D. However, we've already discussed the health problems associated with dairy consumption. Fish oil and dark green leafy vegetables are additional sources. Because of pollution, plant products are preferable over animal products. The sun and dark green leafy vegetables make a great team for providing vitamin D.

In their book entitled *Living Well*, Dale and Kathy Martin list several additional health benefits derived from sunshine, among which are the following:

▶ Aids in losing weight by stimulating the thyroid gland to increase hormone production, thus increasing our rate of metabolism.
▶ Promotes a lowering of blood-sugar levels in the bloodstream, thus giving benefit to diabetics who suffer from too much sugar in their blood.
▶ Promotes the use of oxygen in our tissues.
▶ Tends to improve cardiovascular fitness by helping to reduce blood pressure and decrease cholesterol levels.[4]

Although the sun is an important element to human health, it needs to be taken in proper doses. Excessive exposure to the sun will cause premature aging of the skin, and can lead to skin cancer, the most commonly occurring form of malignancy in America today.[5]

There are three types of skin cancer that have been linked to excessive sun: basal-cell carcinoma, squamous-cell carcinoma, and malignant melanoma. Here are some important facts for you to be aware of:

▶ Every year some 600,000 people are diagnosed with skin cancer. Of these cases 95 percent are basal-cell or squamous-cell carcinomas. The other 5 percent are malignant melanoma.[6]
▶ Basal-cell and squamous-cell are slow-growing cancers, named for the sort of skin cell they originate from.

They tend to be more curable than malignant melanoma.

▶ Malignant melanoma grows fast and is the deadliest form of skin cancer. Between 1973 and 1987 the rate of melanoma increased 83 percent. In comparison, lung cancer dropped by 31.5 percent.[7] Malignant melanoma is the leading cause of cancer in women twenty-five to twenty-nine years of age, and is second only to breast cancer in women thirty to thirty-four.[8]

▶ "Most skin cancers begin in childhood," according to Sydney Hurwitz, M.D., clinical professor of dermatology and pediatrics at the Yale University School of Medicine. Studies reveal that a history of sunburns during the first ten to twenty years of life doubles the risk of skin cancer in later years.[9] Most of us seem to be on the "fry now, pay later" plan when it comes to taking care of our hide during our youth.

▶ The U.S. National Cancer Institute predicts that one out of every six Americans will develop some form of skin cancer in his or her lifetime.[10]

KEY QUOTES

All life on earth requires the sun's energy.
Charles B. Simone, M.D.
Cancer and Nutrition

*So important is sunshine to life
that denying ourselves its life-giving rays
directly contributes to our own undoing.*
Harvey and Marilyn Diamond
Living Health

*Our warm friend is only an enemy to be shunned
if we choose to abuse our bodies by overdoing our exposure
or by consuming a typically high fat diet.
In reality, this ever-present companion is a wonderful*

contributor to our health if we will use it in moderation
and eat a diet which helps our bodies
to effectively utilize the sun's goodness.
Dale and Kathy Martin
Living Health

USE THE SUN WITHOUT ABUSING YOUR BODY

Bathe Your Body, Don't Burn It

There is a big difference between a sunbath and a sunburn. "Sunbathing," observe Harvey and Marilyn Diamond in their book *Living Health*, "is every bit as essential and beneficial as any of the other elements of health, but sunbathe properly!"[11] They suggest that the best time of day to actually bathe your body in sunlight is during the early-morning or late-afternoon hours, and then for only thirty minutes. In the northern hemisphere, the sun is most intense in the summer between the hours of 10:00 a.m. and 3:00 p.m. Avoid sunbathing during these hours.

While taking a sunbath, expose as much skin as possible. In fact, don't even use any sort of sunscreens, oils, or lotions. These actually inhibit the oil-secreting glands of the body from working properly.

Again, it's very important to take your sunbaths during hours when the sun is less intense. As the Diamonds point out, "it is not mere tanning that you are after but a general revitalizing of your entire body that is not confined to the skin alone. . . . When done intelligently in concert with the other elements of health, by taking in the sun you are taking a measure necessary to ensure yourself the highest level of health possible."[12]

Use Sunscreen

It is important that if you're out in intense sun for an extended period of time, you should wear protective clothing and use a sunscreen lotion on unprotected areas of your skin. A longtime standard has been to recommend products with PABA (para-aminobenzoic acid), a B vitamin that absorbs the ultraviolet rays that cause sunburn and skin cancer, and that has a sun-protection factor (SPF) of at least 15. This will block at least 92 percent of ultraviolet rays. Sunscreens with SPF of 30 provide an extra 2 to 3 percent blockage.[13]

Health-food stores are now carrying certain products that may be even better for us than those containing PABA. For instance, octyl methoxycinnate is an organic sunscreen that is reportedly more effective than PABA, and has fewer side effects on the skin. Check out your available options. Bottom line, if you're going to be out in intense sunlight for extended periods of time, get protection. Practice safe sunlight.

Eat Lots of Fruits and Vegetables

Excessive exposure to the sun can cause free radicals to be developed in our skin cells. These are highly destructive molecules that damage tissue, cause premature aging, and can lead to cancer.[14]

If you do spend a significant amount of time out in the sun, add lots of fruits and vegetables to your daily diet. Studies show that these foods, high in carotenes, combat the development of free radicals, raise the threshold at which the sun begins to burn, and increase your tendency to tan instead. As Charles Simone, M.D., suggests, "Eat carrots!"[15]

You should also consider supplementing your diet with vitamins A, C, E, and a mineral called selenium. Along with beta-carotene, these are your most effective allies against free radicals.

Reduce Your Fat Intake

High-fat diets contribute to the aging process of our skin, by creating certain chemical reactions in our bodies referred to as free radicals. These in turn can have a negative impact upon healthy tissue. "Exposure to excessive sunlight intensifies the activity of these rabble rousers to the point that a deranged cell can have its genetic order scrambled and begin to act like someone gone mad."[16] Skin cancer can result.

KEY QUESTION

Q. I want to work on my tan. What about using a tanning booth?

A. It is obvious from my research that most, if not all, health professionals do not condone tanning booths. Here is a sampling of opinion:

James F. Balch, M.D.: "Suntanning beds (those used in tanning salons) were once considered safer than the sun. The equipment in the beds emits only UV-A rays, which are the sun's cool rays. Hot B rays (UV-B) were considered primarily responsible for tanning, burning, and skin cancer. Now there is evidence that the UV-A rays may cause the same damage as the UV-B rays. Beware of tanning salons!"[17]

Michael J. Fransblau, M.D.: "With the development during the past 20 years of high intensity lamps emitting UVA, the suntan facility industry has burgeoned. . . . A growing body of literature indicates the potential for the development of basal and squamous cell carcinomas, as well as the development of cutaneous melanomas on the basis of exposure to UVA. Beginning in the 1980's, it was noted that an increasing number of eye injuries were caused by exposure to UVA in suntan facilities. [Including] Severe burning of the skin, exacerbation of autoimmune illnesses such as lupus erythematosus, photoallergic reactions of the skin, premature aging of the skin, (and) an increase in the number of skin cancers."[18]

Andrew Weil, M.D.: "The popularity of tanning parlors is an indication of widespread ignorance about this matter. The ultraviolet radiation used in them is not safe, no matter what their advertisements say."[19]

Getting sun is an important part of a health-promoting lifestyle. But to be a healthy habit, it must be approached with care. Just as you would not want to take toxic levels of important vitamins or minerals, don't overdose on the sun. Unfortunately, "sun worshiping" is currently prevalent in our culture.

Along with it comes the pressure to have the "perfect tan"—considered a badge of affluence, sex appeal, health, and athleticism. Be careful, very careful, lest you develop the "red badge of cancer."

FURTHER READING

Cancer and Nutrition by Charles B. Simone, M.D. (New York: McGraw-Hill, 1983). See "Light from the Sun—Photolysis," pages 46-49.

Healing Nutrients by Patrick Quillin, Ph.S., R.D. (Chicago: Contemporary Books, 1987). Several discussions throughout the book deal with the importance of vitamin D and calcium.

Living Health by Harvey and Marilyn Diamond (New York: Warner Books, 1987). See chapter 11: "Sunshine."

Living Well by Dale and Kathy Martin (Brentwood, TN: Wolgemuth and Hyatt, 1988). See chapter 8: "Outward Bound—Fresh Air, Sunshine, and Exercise."

18
BREATHE CLEAN AIR

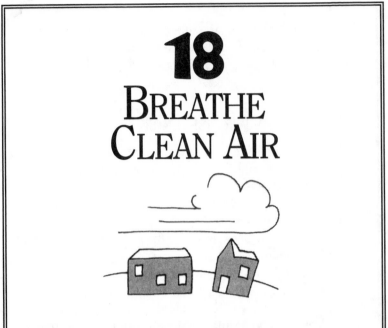

Air is *the* most important nutrient for human life. You and I have been designed by our Creator to run on oxygen. Every day we take over 17,000 breaths that serve to keep our bodies fueled with this precious gas. Every cell in our system requires it in order to remain healthy and to properly contribute to our bodies.

WHY BREATHE CLEAN AIR?

The earth is currently home to about 6,000 billion tons of air.[1] Quantity-wise, we're doing fine. Quality, however, is another story. If you're concerned about staying healthy, it's time to think about what kind of air you're feeding yourself.

Pollution (Outdoors)
Much of the air we breathe outdoors is dirty. Here are some "breathtaking" facts:

▶ According to the American Lung Association, 164 million U.S. citizens (two-thirds of our population) breathe air that the Environmental Protection Agency (EPA) considers unhealthy.[2]

▶ In the Los Angeles area, for instance, air pollution fall-out amounts to 10 million pounds a day—cough, gag![3]

Pollution (Indoors)

The EPA considers indoor air pollution one of the top environmental problems of the 1990s.

Pollution levels—According to Ron White, senior program manager for the American Lung Association's Air Conservation and Occupational Health Program, "Typical indoor levels of pollutants can be up to 20 times higher than outdoor levels."[4] Also, tests done by the EPA confirm that indoor levels of toxic chemical pollution are much greater than outdoor pollution, even in our biggest cities.[5]

Related medical costs—In 1989 the EPA issued a report in which they estimated that eight of the most common indoor air pollutants cost the nation more than $1 billion in medical costs from cancer and heart disease.[6]

Toxic chemicals—The products found in average American households across the country contain a combined total of some 63,000 different chemicals. Many of these chemicals are toxic, becoming more so as they interact with each other inside a closed environment.[7]

Formaldehyde—is a toxic chemical widely used in building products and household goods as a bonding agent and preservative. Many pressed-wood products such as plywood, particle board, paneling, cabinets, furniture, and countertops contain this chemical. So do some shampoos, lipsticks, toothpastes, eye makeups, perfumes, hairsprays, nail polishes, soaps, toilet tissue, milk cartons, car bodies, household disinfectants, curtains, carpets, upholstery fabrics, linens, and insulation. "Formaldehyde puts the 'permanent' in permanent press clothing and the 'strength' in wet-strength paper towels."[8]

Radon—A naturally occurring radioactive gas, radon may be contaminating as many as 10 percent of the homes in the United States. In some parts of the country, this number may be higher. It is a colorless, odorless gas produced by the breakdown of uranium in rock and soil. It enters structures through cracks in their foundations, and unless somehow dispersed, can lead to lung damage and cancer. In fact, radon is second only to smoking as a leading cause of lung cancer. The National Cancer Institute estimates that radon causes 20,000 to 30,000 deaths a year.[9]

Tobacco smoke—Tobacco smoke is a common indoor pollutant. Every year about 467,000 tons of tobacco are burned indoors, based upon the fact that Americans spend 90 percent of their time indoors, and smoke annual totals of 600 billion cigarettes, 4 billion cigars, and 11 billion pipefuls of tobacco.[10]

Leaded paint—Leaded paint may be a problem in most homes built before 1950. In fact, the U.S. Department of Housing and Urban Development (HUD) suspects that 74 percent of all private dwellings built before 1980 have some amount of lead paint on their walls. If lead dust is inhaled, it can cause significant cellular damage and a host of health problems.[11]

Associated Health Problems
Polluted air has been associated with a number of health problems, including:

lung cancer	headaches
cardiovascular disease	cramps
leukemia	irritation of eyes, ears, nose,
nausea	throat, lungs, and sinuses
dizziness	fatigue
skin rashes	drowsiness
persistent cough	insomnia
joint and muscle pain	mental confusion
incoherent speech	memory loss
depression	sudden infant death syndrome (SIDS)

KEY QUOTES

Of all the elements available for sustaining us,
air is probably the one most taken for granted. Yet 17,000
involuntary breaths daily can hardly

be counted as insignificant.
Dale and Kathy Martin
Living Well

It is possible to go weeks without food and days without water, but six minutes without air and you're a corpse.
Harvey Diamond
Living Health

HOW TO BREATHE CLEAN AIR

The question is, what can you do as an individual to take control of your environment and help ensure the quality of the air you breathe? When it comes to outdoor air, that's difficult. So much is beyond your individual control. There are a few things you can do to make sure that you're not adding to outdoor pollution—things like keeping your car well tuned and effectively burning fuel, driving less, switching your fireplace from wood to gas. If you exercise outdoors, you can decide to do so in the early morning, when the air is clearest and the cars have not begun to pile up pollutants in the neighborhood. You could also pick up your belongings and move away from the city or the industry or the "whatever" that's nearby adding pollutants to your air.

There is another area in which you can extend more personal control over the air you breathe, and that is in your home. As was mentioned earlier, one of the biggest problems of the 1990s is indoor air pollution. Already 63,000 different chemicals are found in homes across the nation in various manufactured products. Every day 1,000 new ones are invented.[12] Since the average American spends 90 percent of his or her time indoors, and much of that is at home, your dwelling represents a very important place to begin to make some changes. Here are just a few simple ones to get you started on your road toward breathing cleaner and easier in the most important of places, your home.

Keep Your Dwelling Well Ventilated

Airtight living spaces are great for conserving energy in the winter months, but they provide an environment in which pollutants accumulate. Crack a window or a door each day and let in fresh air. If you own your own home, you might consider installing a system called a heat-recovery ventilator, also known as an air-to-air heat exchanger. It draws outdoor air into the house and recovers the heat from the indoor air before exhausting it to the outside.[13] But for most of us, the most cost-effective thing we can do is simply air out the house once a day.

Bedrooms are especially important areas of the home to keep well ventilated. We spend about one-third of our lives in them. It is suggested that they be aired out each day, and that a window be cracked at night, even in the coldest of climes.

Use Nontoxic Household Cleaning Products

A gallon of water mixed with ¼ cup of white vinegar and a teaspoon of baking soda makes a good all-purpose cleaner. If it's windows you're doing, just leave out the baking soda (¼ cup white vinegar + one quart water). If you're scouring the sink, leave out the vinegar and add more baking soda to make a paste. If it's the sink drain that needs some attention, try unclogging it with a mixture of ¼ cup baking soda, ½ cup vinegar, and boiling water.

Check at your local natural-foods store for additional safe household products. Some supermarkets are now carrying lines of products that are more environmentally safe, as well. Look for products that are "biodegradable" and free of phosphates, petroleum, hydrochloric acid, sulfuric acid, benzene, and chlorine.

For a host of other ideas on how to buy or make your own nontoxic household cleaners, pick up one of the books listed below.

Keep Your Furnace, Humidifier, and Air Conditioner Clean

Whatever sorts of mechanisms you have in your house that impact the quality of your air should be regularly serviced and cleaned, and the filters should be changed. Check into having your air ducts professionally cleaned, as well.

Ban Smoking
We've already seen the effects of smoke, both to the smoker and to the innocent bystander. If you haven't already read the chapter "Quit Smoking," please do so.

Get Your Place Checked for Radon
For testing information contact your regional office of the Environmental Protection Agency (EPA) or write:

EPA Public Information Center
401 M Street SW
Washington, DC 20460
(202) 260-2080

Fortunately, if you've got a radon problem, it can be taken care of fairly easily. So don't put it off.

Get a Lead-Testing Kit
For about $25.00 you can test the paint in your home. You can get a kit by writing or calling one of the following companies:

Frandon Enterprises	Hybrivet Systems	Seventh Generation
511 N. 48th Street	P.O. Box 1210	49 Hercules Drive
Seattle, WA 98103	Framingham, MA 01701	Colchester, VT 05446
(800)359-9000	(800)262-LEAD	(800)456-1177
(416)293-4955	(508)651-7881	

A couple named Donald and Frances Wallace run Frandon Enterprises. Their story is that a few years back they both nearly died from lead poisoning. Seems they had begun to display a number of troubling symptoms of something gone awry, but exactly what remained a mystery. Their list of health problems steadily mounted: insomnia, anemia, dehydration, severe abdominal cramps, sudden attacks of total body pain, weight loss, personality change, nervous system dysfunction, and flulike symptoms. It appeared to some medical authorities like Alzheimer's disease was setting in. To others, some of the pains Mr. Wallace was experiencing in particular seemed related to carpal tunnel syndrome.

Finally, after several misdiagnoses and unnecessary operations, their self-diagnosis of chronic lead poisoning was confirmed by doctors. Seems they'd purchased some mugs during a vacation in Italy several years earlier, and had been drinking a good eight to ten cups of coffee from them on a daily basis for over three years. Come to find, the cups contained lead in their construction and were giving off four hundred times more than the Food and Drug Administration (FDA) considers within safe limits.[14]

The moral of the story is that it's not just your paint you need to be concerned about.

Decorate with Lots of Plants

People take in oxygen and give off carbon dioxide. Plants absorb carbon dioxide and produce oxygen. One species' trash is another's treasure. Plants are a wonderful way to help keep your indoor air clean, besides adding life and color to your decor. An especially crucial area of your home to use plants would be in your bedroom, where a lot of carbon dioxide can accumulate each night.

FURTHER READING

Diet for a Poisoned Planet by David Steinman (New York: Harmony Books, 1990). See chapter 15: "The Nontoxic Home."

Everyday Cancer Risks and How to Avoid Them by Mary Kerney Levenstein (Garden City Park, NY: Avery Publishing Group, 1992). See chapter 16: "Indoor Pollution and Household Products"; chapter 23: "Radon"; chapter 13: "Formaldehyde"; chapter 33: "Smoking—Active and Passive."

Healthy Homes in a Toxic World by Maury M. Breecher,

M.P.H., and Shirley Linde, Ph.D. (New York: John Wiley
and Sons, 1992). See chapter 2: "Radon Gas—A Deadly
Threat to Millions"; chapter 3: "Indoor Air Pollution—
The Enemy Within"; chapter 4: "Revitalizing Indoor
Air—Ventilation and Air Cleaning." And many more
important chapters.

Living Health by Harvey and Marilyn Diamond (New York:
Warner Books, 1987). See chapter 6: "Air."

The Non-Toxic Home by Debra Lynn Dadd (Los Angeles:
Jeremy P. Tarcher, 1986). Ideas concerning protecting
your family from toxins and health hazards.

19

EFFECTIVELY DEAL WITH NEGATIVE STRESS

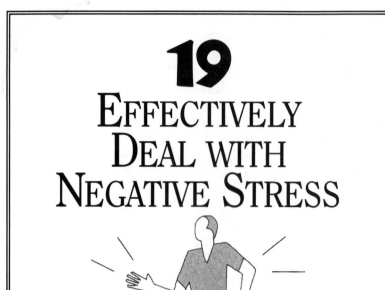

Our lives are filled with different kinds and intensities of stress. Some we perceive as positive—winning the lottery and being faced with what to do with 2.7 million dollars, for instance. Most of us would volunteer readily to see if we couldn't find ways to successfully handle that sort of stress. Falling in love, getting married, buying a home, giving birth to a child—these are more examples of potentially positive forms of stress that we willingly allow into our lives with feelings of hope and fulfillment.

Then there's that *other* kind of stress. Like when you receive notice from Uncle Sam that your tax return is about to be audited, or your spouse calls to tell you that the car's just been towed to Larry's Car Barn because something under the hood caught on fire, or your child decides that it's time to paint his room with a magic marker. These kinds of stressors, which no doubt most of us would consider negative, have a way of keeping our lives from becoming a sea of tranquility.

Finally, some of us suffer under long-term negative stress, sometimes referred to as chronic stress. This kind of stress is characterized day in and day out by circumstances we perceive as unpleasant. For example, many consider the constant pressure they're under in their jobs a form of chronic negative stress.

WHY DEAL WITH STRESS?

Whether we like it or not, stress, both positive and negative, is a part of human existence. Health professionals are warning us, however, that if we want to live long and healthy lives, we must learn how to deal effectively and constructively with negative stress. Some reasons follow.

Cancer

Studies done by researchers at the University of Texas point to the conclusion that when our brains are under negative stress, they manufacture an excess amount of a hormone called ACTH. This hormone inhibits our body's production of white blood cells, which make up our immune system and are vital for warding off disease.[1] Cancer is a disease of a weakened immune system.

Heart Attacks, Strokes, and Nervous Breakdowns

It all starts as the body's stores of vitamins and minerals are drained. Vitamin C reserves are the first to come under attack during stressful periods. Huge amounts of B vitamins, A, E, and pantothenic acid are used up as well. As the stores of calcium, magnesium, phosphorus, and potassium are also depleted, your body draws replacement minerals from bones, teeth, hair, organs, and other tissues to meet the demands. Under stress the stomach also slows down its production of hydrochloric acid. When this happens protein metabolism becomes impaired. Bottom line, you're losing more nutrients than you're able to replace. You're on your way to a complete health breakdown of some kind.

In his book *Lazy Person's Guide to Better Nutrition,* Gordon S. Tessler, Ph.D., observes: "As the body becomes deficient in essential nutrients, its ability to resist the stressors diminishes. If a stress is prolonged for weeks, months or years, the body is unable to convert cholesterol into needed hormones. Such continued stress results in complete exhaustion and total collapse."[2] Heart attacks, strokes, and "nervous breakdowns" are examples of what happens to a body completely drained by stress.

Other Health Problems
In his book *Coronary? Cancer? God's Answer: Prevent It!*, author and medical doctor Richard Brennan points out that "emotional stress causes or aggravates disorders of the digestive system, the circulatory system, the genito-urinary system, the nervous system, and the glands of internal secretion, as well as causing allergic disorders, muscle-joint disorders, infections, and eye and skin disease."[3]

More specifically, these system disorders include things like high blood pressure, migraine headaches, neckaches, ulcers, diarrhea, colitis, irritable bowels, constipation, dizziness, depression, respiratory infections, and allergies.

KEY QUOTES

Research is increasingly finding that our thoughts, attitudes, feelings, and philosophies play a major role in keeping us well, or producing illness.
Mike Samuels, M.D.
The Well Adult

There is not a single cell of the body totally removed from the influence of mind and emotions.
The British Medical Society

The unresolvable stress overload is the cause of many illnesses and deaths in the United States.
Gordon S. Tessler, Ph.D.
Lazy Person's Guide to Better Nutrition

*Stress is one of the most powerful, and most insidious,
factors that can hurt your immune system.*
Stuart M. Berger, M.D.
Dr. Berger's Immune Power Diet

HOW TO DEAL WITH STRESS

Obviously, eliminating all forms of negative stress from our lives is simply not possible. Life just doesn't work that way. However, you and I can do some very practical things to help ourselves deal more effectively and constructively with life's not-so-positive circumstances. We don't need to play helpless victim, letting negative situations have their way with our health. Dr. Nancy Appleton points out that "it's not life's situations, but how we deal with them, which determines whether we let stress become distress."[4]

What follows are ten ways to keep stress from becoming distress.

Recognize Stress

Spend some time trying to isolate and identify the major sources of negative stress in your life. Ask and answer the simple question, "What's bothering me?" Make a list. Give yourself plenty of time to get in touch with the various areas in your life where negative stressors may be "eating" on you. It's hard to fight an enemy you can't quite identify. The following categories may help you to unlock specific areas of stress:

marital problems	child-raising problems
financial difficulties	pressures at work
too many commitments	lack of career direction
lack of purpose in life	feelings of social isolation
lack of acceptance from others	

Talk About Stress

Find a trusted friend or a group of such friends with whom you can be open and honest concerning these areas of negative stress. Dr. Mike Samuels observes that "support is the functional opposite of stress."[5] He lists the following reasons why social support increases health:

- ▶ It gratifies emotional needs for security, affection, trust, intimacy, nurturing, and a sense of belonging.
- ▶ It helps in appraising and defining reality.
- ▶ It makes people aware of shared norms of feeling and behavior.
- ▶ It increases group solidarity.
- ▶ It increases self-esteem through social approval.

Turn to God for His Help and Peace

As part of helping people cope with stress better, Dr. Tessler says, "I am a firm believer in the need for human beings to spend time in religious and spiritual pursuits. . . . Take time to make a connection with the source of your life and be thankful for all your Creator has given you."[6]

Abraham Lincoln, no stranger to stress, was one who shared Dr. Tessler's view on the importance of connecting with God. It was during his administration as President of the United States that the whole country erupted into a self-destructive civil war. Of that tumultuous time in his life, Lincoln has said: "Amid the greatest difficulties of my Administration, when I could not see any other resort, I would place my whole reliance in God." Later, when a delegation presented him with a Bible, he replied: "This great book is the best gift God has given to man. But for it we could not know right from wrong."[7]

Envision Yourself in Control

Researchers have found that people who have learned to see themselves as helplessly trapped in their circumstances are more likely than others to develop disease. "People, and even animals," writes Dr. Samuels, "who believe that their actions have no effect on the outcome of a situation—that they have no control over their world—are more prone to illness."[8] On the other hand, those who practice seeing themselves in control over their situation reduce the negative effects of stress. By envisioning the power to make changes, you're sending health-promoting messages to your body.

My wife and I experienced the importance of this mental attitude in our own battle with cancer (see Introduction to this book), a very stressful situation, indeed. Had we agreed with the doctors that Anne was little more than a helpless victim to the disease, we would've been overwhelmed with distress. As it was, we took control of the strategy, much like a commander in the midst of a battlefield, and won back her health.

Set Goals for Managing Stress

Make and begin to work toward short- and long-term goals in each of the areas of most significant negative stress to you. Because the joy of success breeds more success, start your changes with the areas of stress that you find the easiest to deal with.

Find Sources of Help

If you need it, get outside help that will enable you to move forward toward your goals. For instance, if you have money problems, you may want to consult with a professional financial advisor. If you're experiencing parenting problems, maybe a family counselor could help you with better strategies for raising your children. There are professionals available to help you in every area of your life.

Exercise Daily

Exercise is a wonderful stress reducer. Some find that morning exercise helps to prepare them to handle the hassles of the day. Others prefer evening exercise as a form of winding down. Either way, exercise is vitally important to your body's ability to withstand negative stress. As we saw in an earlier chapter, exercise lowers blood pressure, strengthens the heart, oxygenates your cells, and improves your spirit. Studies have shown that those who exercise regularly feel more capable and confident of overcoming the negatives setbacks in life.

"It is an amazing concept that exercise can help 'tune' the body to cope with stress," observes Dr. Samuels. "And it is particularly pertinent, and important, to men and women today whose health patterns are so greatly affected by stress."[9]

Get the Rest You Need

Quite simply, lack of sleep decreases our resistance to stress. Problems always seem smaller following a good night's rest.

Eat Healthy

Follow the dietary suggestions already presented in this book. What we feed our bodies does determine in large measure how they handle the effects of emotional stress. "Eating patterns can be modified in order to help a person cope with the stress of modern day living," writes Gordon Tessler. "A body in optimum health is prepared for stress and able to respond with the needed energy to cope with life."[10]

Develop Hobbies or Other Relaxing Activities

Find something you really enjoy doing that will remove your mind from your problems periodically. Dr. Tessler predicts that "the doctor of the future will prescribe one hour a day of play to reduce stress and improve health."[11]

In the midst of our own busy schedules, my wife and I set aside part of one school day each week (usually Fridays) which we call "play day." More often than not we head down to the Goodwill store to hunt for bargains and treasures. We find it physically relaxing, emotionally restorative, and mentally stimulating.

Here's another approach you might consider for handling stress, offered by David Steenblock, D.O. He calls it the "Steenblock Stress Reduction Plan."

1. List *all* your problems.
2. List *all* possible solutions to each problem. (Take your time. Spend one to two days. Let your imagination run wild.)

3. Quantify the solutions.

IDEA	PRO'S	CON'S
1	4 POINTS	6 POINTS
2	3 POINTS	5 POINTS
3	8 POINTS	3 POINTS
4	9 POINTS	1 POINT

4. Determine from exercise 3 the appropriate solutions to each problem, or recognize that you can't do anything about the problem.
5. Plan a course of action to solve each problem based on your answers to 4. Your action plan should be a well-thought-out, practical, day-by-day, hour-by-hour approach. There should also be an acceptance on your part concerning those problems for which you can do nothing.

FURTHER READING

Everyday Cancer Risks and How to Avoid Them by Mary Kerney Levenstein (Garden City Park, NY: Avery Publishing Group, 1992). See chapter 34: "Stress."

Lazy Person's Guide to Better Nutrition by Gordon S. Tessler, Ph.D. (San Diego: Better Health Publishers, 1984). See chapter 10: "Stress—How to Cope."

Stress Without Distress by Hans Selye, M.D. (New York: The New American Library, 1974).

The Well Adult by Mike Samuels, M.D., and Nancy Samuels (New York: Summit Books, 1988). See chapter 3: "Stress and Health."

20
PLAN "FAST" DAYS

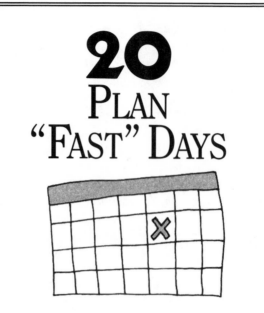

A man's wife passed away after a lengthy illness. The widower was so distraught and unwilling to live life without her that he determined to end it all. One morning he got up, left a suicide note, and hiked up into the mountains. Convinced he could simply starve himself to death, he merely took occasional drinks from the mountain streams to quench his thirst. Weeks passed and the bereaved widower noticed that although he had lost some weight, he was not any nearer death. In fact, he had never felt better in his life. Many ailments he'd suffered from for years had simply disappeared. After a month the man descended from the mountain, looking years younger. He eventually remarried, sired several children, and raised a family.

THE PHYSICAL BENEFITS OF FASTING

It's a proven fact that one of the most health-promoting habits we can develop is that of periodic fasting. I put this chapter last in the book, however, because fasting is the thing that most of us would choose to do least. To fast means to abstain from food. Fluids are taken—sometimes freshly made juices, sometimes just water. Throughout history people have fasted to maintain good health, to draw closer to God, to shed unwanted pounds, to reverse degenerative diseases, and even as a means of protest (known as a hunger strike). Hippocrates, Paracelsus, Galen, and all the other great physicians of old prescribed fasting and considered it "the greatest remedy; the physician within."[1]

Here are some specific benefits you can enjoy through fasting.

Internal Purging and Healing

Fasting gives the body a break from the hard work of digestion in order to redirect some of its energy toward cleaning and healing. During a prolonged fast (after the first three days), we begin to burn and digest our own tissues—a self-digestion process known as autolysis. But, this does not happen indiscriminately! Because of the healing wisdom that God has programed into our bodies, they first feed themselves on those cells and tissues which are diseased, damaged, aged, or dead.[2] Thus fasting helps our bodies to "clean up their acts."

When my wife sought out the advice of a nutritionist for help against her cancer, the very first thing suggested was a juice fast—nothing but freshly made juices for two solid weeks. We thought she was crazy. Who'd ever heard of such a thing! But as we began to learn more about fasting and the body's incredible God-given ability to heal itself if given the right circumstances, we began to understand. In the end, the juice fast was a key part of a very successful cancer battle plan. As Allan Cott, M.D., explains in his book *Fasting as a Way of Life*, "Fasting does not cure chronic diseases or anything else, but it has helped the body to heal itself of more distresses than we may dream."[3]

Cellular Rebuilding and Rejuvenation

In another book entitled *How to Keep Slim, Healthy, and Young with Juice Fasting*, Paavo Airola, N.D., Ph.D., observes: "During fasting, while the old cells and disease tissues are decomposed and burned, the building of new healthy cells is stimulated and speeded up."[4] In other words, fasting not only burns away a lot of the decaying debris in our systems that leads to health problems, but helps in the process of building new cells. As old cells are being decomposed, their amino acids are released and resynthesized to help form the proteins of which new cells are made.

Modification or Elimination of Addictions

Dr. Cott tells of the success of several of his patients who were able to quit smoking as a result of doing five- to six-day fasts. "None reported withdrawal symptoms or any desire to return to smoking. Fasting succeeded where all the New Year's resolutions and other efforts to stop smoking had failed."[5]

Others of his patients who were problem drinkers also found that fasting, for even just one week, helped them to significantly alter their alcohol habits.

Other Benefits

Fasting can also be beneficial for the following:

   weight loss
   increased energy levels
   improved mental powers
   rejuvenated nervous system
   normalized chemistry in tissues
   revitalized functioning of glands and organs
   improved digestion and utilization of nutrients

WHY I LIKE TO FAST

Anne Frähm
Physically, I feel great after an extended fast. I have more energy, my skin is notably softer and clearer, and I feel amazingly light. I've lost some weight and reduced that bloated "all over" feeling. Mentally, I feel good about myself because I know I've done something good for my body. I've gotten rid of stored up toxins and accumulated "gunk," my mind is clearer, and I have

the deep-down satisfaction that comes from exercising self-control. I've noticed that when I take control over the desires of my fleshly body, it gives me more control in other areas of my life. As an added bonus, I can wear ALL of my clothes!

Dave Frähm
I'd have to say ditto to all that Anne has mentioned. I would also add that fasting always has a way of drawing me closer to God. It's kind of hard to explain, but when I go without food for a few days and begin to break my daily reliance and focus upon it, I begin to see and experience God in a whole new light. Well, not entirely new. Both Anne and I are Christians who firmly believe that God is our provider. But it's just that while fasting, the reality of God as provider seems so much more vivid. Like going from black and white to color. Somehow my sense of God's presence and my complete reliance upon him are heightened when I'm fasting.

KEY QUOTES

Fasting is the most efficient means of correcting any disease.
Adolph Mayer, M.D.

Thousands of people throughout the world fast regularly
not to cure any particular disease,
but because they consider fasting to be an effective way
to cleanse the body from accumulated wastes,
build up the physical stamina and resistance against disease,
and revitalize and rejuvenate the functions
of all their vital organs.
Paavo O. Airola, N.D., Ph.D.

Fasting does not cure chronic diseases or anything else,
but it has helped the body to heal itself
of more distresses than we may dream.
Alan Cott, M.D.
Fasting as a Way of Life

*Fasting is . . . a royal road to healing for anyone who agrees
to take it for the recovery and regeneration of the body.*
Otto H. F. Buchinger, M.D.

HOW TO FAST

It's simple: stop eating. Technically, a fast involves consumption of water only. However, the juice fast is considered superior by many health professionals. Their contention is that fasting on freshly made juices of fruits and vegetables, plus vegetable broths and herb teas, "results in much faster recovery from disease and more effective cleansing and rejuvenation of the tissues than does the traditional water fast."[6]

In 1992, the juicer was the biggest selling small appliance in the United States. Hopefully these machines are not simply gathering dust on the shelves of America's pantries. The concentrated vitamins, minerals, amino acids, and enzymes our bodies can use from freshly made fruit and vegetable juices are limitless. Dilute your freshly pressed juices with equal parts of pure water and consume within ten minutes, if possible. Fresh juices can be preserved fairly well for a few hours in a vacuum-sealed thermos bottle if necessary.

Some juicers are better than others. We enjoy using a Champion brand juicer, well known for its ability to preserve the quality of the nutrients released during the juicing process. Check at your local health-food store for juicers and organic produce.

When fasting, it is important to do three things:

Drink a Lot!
Dr. Cott recommends drinking at least two quarts of liquid daily. It aids in eliminating toxins from the body. Select from any of the following as often as you want:

Fruit juice*	Vegetable broth
Herb tea	Vegetable juice
Purified water (with a squeeze of lemon)	

(*Some people with special health concerns like hypo-glycemia or candida may not be able to tolerate the concentrated amounts of simple sugars in fruit juices. Please consult with a nutritional specialist.)

Do Enemas and Colonics

Enemas are the gentle flushing of the colon (large intestine), accomplished by introducing water through a device inserted into the rectum. Doing these while fasting helps to remove toxins from the body. Dr. Airola explains:

> The main purpose of fasting is to help the body to cleanse itself from accumulated toxic wastes. By the process of autolysis, a huge amount of morbid matter, dead cells and diseased tissues are burned; and the toxic wastes which have accumulated in the tissues for years, causing disease and premature aging, are loosened and expelled from the system. The alimentary canal (colon) . . . is the main road by which these toxins are thrown out of the body. Since, during fasting, the natural bowel movements cease to take place, the toxic wastes would have no way of leaving the system, except with the help of enemas and colonics.[7]

Colonics, sometimes referred to as colon irrigations, are glorified enemas. They involve several flushings over a period of time (typically an hour), administered by a trained technician using a machine that is specially designed for the purpose. The water flow (several gallons administered a pint or two at a time) and expulsion are controlled by the technician and machine.

The concept of colon cleansing for health reasons has been around for thousands of years. As early as 2500 BC there were "bowel specialists" in the Egyptian society.[8] Both enemas and colonics serve to help flush released toxins from your body. While a colonic is something you need to see a specialist for (unless, of course, you just happen to own a colonic machine), enemas are self-administered in your home.

You can purchase an enema kit at most drugstores. It comes with a hot-water bottle and hook, a hose that attaches to the bottle with a clamp to adjust flow, and a tip that screws onto the hose and is inserted into the rectum.

Here are the steps to go through when giving yourself an enema:

1. Fluid preparation
   ▶ Warm eight cups of distilled (or otherwise purified) water to body temperature.
2. Kit preparation
   ▶ Find a place in or near your bathroom where you can lie down and suspend the hot-water bottle about twelve inches above you.
   ▶ Fill the bottle with the water.
   ▶ Screw hose to bottle and tip to hose.
   ▶ Allow a trickle of water to escape before clamping hose, in order to get rid of air in the line.
   ▶ Apply lubricant to the tip. (Aloe Vera gel works great.)
3. Body preparation
   ▶ Lie down on your left side with your hips elevated (use small pillow covered with plastic bag, put towel over this).
   ▶ Insert tip carefully into rectum. (Takes practice. Be gentle. Don't get discouraged if it's not easy at first.)
4. Flow
   ▶ Adjust flow to comfort.
   ▶ Take in as much as comfortable (massaging abdomen from left to right).
   ▶ Clamp hose before removing tip from rectum.
   ▶ Lie on your back, then on your right side—two to three minutes each.
   ▶ Expel into toilet, massaging abdomen from right to left.
5. Clean up
   ▶ Rinse hot-water bottle, hose, tip, and plastic cover on pillow.

- ▶ Sterilize bathroom surfaces with disinfectant (toilet stool, floor, etc.).
- ▶ Put tip in liquid bleach, washing with HOT water before using again.

Special note: Because enemas tend to wash out the good bacteria in the colon along with everything else, it is important to consume several doses a day of a live bacteria culture known as "acidophilus" to help restore your own natural intestinal flora. Follow manufacturer's recommendations on the label as far as how much to take and when. Potassium that is lost during enemas is restored via consumption of vegetable broths.

Break a Fast Gently
Dr. Airola states, "Breaking a fast is the most significant phase of it. The beneficial effect of fasting could be totally undone if the fast is broken incorrectly."[9] He recommends several days of gradual transition to the normal diet. For example, the first day following a fast the menu might consist of an apple and a small salad, in addition to the juices. He stresses to be careful not to overeat and to chew your food extremely well.

KEY QUESTIONS

Q. How often should one fast?

A. Many people like to fast one day a week. Others like to go for three to ten days every three months. When Anne had cancer she juice-fasted for two weeks. Now she does periodic three- to five-day fasts to clean out her body and maintain good health. There are no "set in cement" rules for how often one should fast or for how long. Listen to your body. As you become more aware of its signals, you will know when your system needs to take time off from digestion for a good cleaning.

Q. Are there any side effects I should anticipate while fasting?

A. Yes, during a fast your body switches from a sustaining, maintenance mode to a "dumping" and detoxification mode.

You'll be using up energy for elimination rather than digestion. Your eliminative organs—liver, kidneys, colon, skin, and lungs—will be working hard to "clean house." You'll know this is taking place when your breath and body odor begin to smell putrid, your tongue is coated, and you're experiencing skin eruptions. You may alternate between feeling dizzy, headachy, weak, and flulike to euphoric and energetic. Generally, the more toxic you are to begin with, the worse you will feel initially. In the words of Rudolph Ballentine, M.D., "Cleansing is most unpleasant when it is overdue."[10] Keep in mind your goal—a clean, rejuvenated body.

Q. How active can I be while I'm on a fast?

A. The answer to that question is totally up to you. Our bodies and our lifestyles are all different. There is no standard answer. Some people are able to maintain their usual routine while fasting. Others find it important to cut way back on their activities.

The nutritionist who helped Anne battle back from cancer does a fast every Monday as she carries on her daily routine. Another friend sets aside one weekend every two months to do a fast. Some people use their vacations to go to health resorts where they can fast outside the boundaries of their daily routine. Bottom line, do what works best for you. Design your own program.

FURTHER READING

Fasting as a Way of Life by Allan Cott, M.D. (New York: Bantam Books, 1977).

How to Keep Slim, Healthy, and Young with Juice Fasting by Paavo O. Airola, N.D., Ph.D. (Phoenix, AZ: Health Plus Publishers, 1971).

Juicing for Life by Cherie Calbom and Maureen Keane (Garden City Park, NY: Avery Publishing Group, 1992).

Raw Vegetable Juices by Norman W. Walker, Ph.D. (Phoenix, AZ: Norwalk Press Publishers, 1936).

QUESTIONS AND ANSWERS

Q. If I travel or just eat out a lot, how can I effectively maintain a health-promoting diet?

A. Here are some tips:

1. Try patronizing vegetarian restaurants.

2. At regular restaurants, look for their vegetarian entrees. More and more restaurants are adding these to their menus in response to a growing number of requests. If no strictly vegetarian meals are served, ask for double helpings of potatoes, vegetables, beans, or grains in lieu of the meat. Many establishments will accommodate you in this way.

3. Wherever you eat, look for foods that contain no dairy, no meat, low salt, low oil (fat). Avoid the dessert page of the menu.

4. Make veggie salads part of lunch and dinner. Ask for low-fat dressing, or go with vinegar and a bit of olive oil. Lemon juice is also very good. Even some fast-food restaurants are now offering salad bars. Just be careful not to load up on high-fat salad dressing. If nothing else

is available, go without the dressing or bring your own.

5. Hot or cold cereals for breakfast are good. Avoid using the milk. If you go with toast, ask for unbuttered whole-wheat. Many restaurants also offer fruit plates. These are a good choice, but be sure not to eat fruit with other foods.

6. If you're flying somewhere and want to make sure you maintain your health-supporting diet, ask for vegetarian meals when you make your reservations. Bring along your own drinking water—many people do. If you really want to be prepared, bring your own food and avoid the airline stuff altogether.

Q. What if I'm invited to somebody's house for a meal? How can I be an enjoyable, unoffensive guest without at the same time offending my body?

A. There are several things you can do. Choose those options that seem best in light of the relationship you enjoy and how things will be taken. Make your friendship the primary issue, and food secondary. Here are some ideas:

1. When invited, explain up front that you're on a special diet for health reasons which precludes meat and dairy. Tell them what you can eat—salads with low-fat dress-ing, potatoes, legumes, grains, whole-grain breads, soups, steamed vegetables—and see if they'd still like you to join them. This up-front approach is usually the best.

2. If you're invited over for the ever-popular barbecue, ask if it's okay if you bring your own meat substitute. Explain that you're on a special diet for health reasons. Take along your soy-dogs and soy-burgers.

3. Another option is to simply show up and eat whatever they're serving. Count this as your one "feast meal" of the week. Remember, it's not what you eat 5 percent of the time that'll do you harm, but the food you feed your body the other 95 percent of the time. Even so, practice a certain amount of restraint. You can easily pass up cer-tain things, dessert for instance, without offending.

4. If you're going to be staying in another person's home

for a time, be very sure to explain up front your dietary needs and constraints. Offer to get involved in food purchase and preparation. More often than not, your hosts will become intrigued by the information you're sharing and will want to find out all they can about your new eating habits. Everyone is concerned about health. Teach but don't preach. Keep it "I" centered. Share things you've learned that have helped you be healthier. Don't start telling them what they should do unless they open that door.

Q. What if guests are coming to my house?

A. That's simple. Put together your very best and most tasty vegetarian meal or menu of meals, depending on how long they're staying. Use the opportunity to help others see just how inviting and delicious a meal can be, even without meat and dairy products. Your friends are entering your world, so explain it to them a bit. Dietary things need not take up the entire conversation around the dinner table, but your friends will undoubtedly be interested in learning more about your personal "culture," just as they would when visiting another country. Again, teach but don't preach.

Q. Will maintaining a health-promoting diet cost me more for food than the diet we Americans typically tend to eat?

A. It has been our experience that at first it will. You'll find yourself in a transitional period for awhile in which you're being reeducated about food and health. It's almost like going back to school. You'll begin to realize just how many products you have in your kitchen that should not be consumed. The wisest thing you can do with them is to simply throw them out. Giving them to a friend or relative would not be doing them any favors. In the process of creating your own new "food culture," you'll be experimenting, trying new things. This will cost money. Consider it money well spent toward your unofficial doctorate in health and nutrition.

Once you've learned your way through the bulk of this transitional period of building your own new culture, you will discover that your food cost will drop. Even if you're only cutting back on meat and dairy products, and you still eat a few processed foods, these are your high-cost items. If you take the most health-promoting route and drop these products altogether, you'll see real money savings.

In all of this it's also important to take a long-term view of things. Going this way with your eating habits will potentially save you lots and lots of money in health-care costs—a topic that is at the very top of most personal, corporate, and governmental agendas these days.

Q. This book is written to help me take personal responsibility for my health. Suppose somewhere along the line I do need the help of professionals. To whom should I turn?

A. We recommend that you begin to develop a network of resources upon whom you can call for specific health-related issues. Many people have a family doctor, quite often an M.D. or D.O. (Doctor of Osteopathy). We suggest that you also add to your resource list the following:

▶ *Certified Nutritionist or Naturopathic Doctor (N.D.)*—A professional who can help you with diet, nutrition, and defense against degenerative disease. There are some M.D.'s and D.O.'s who are using more and more nutritional therapies in their practices. These are "rare birds," however. Most traditionally trained physicians have no background in preventative medicine.

▶ *Chiropractor*—A professional who can help you maintain the structural integrity of your human machine. Pinched nerves, misalignment of the spine, and other structural infirmities can lead to even greater health problems down the line if left untended. Getting and keeping your structural systems in good repair is also an important part of long-term disease prevention.

Q. What about taking dietary supplements?

A. In the June 7, 1993, edition of *Newsweek* magazine, one of the major stories was entitled "Vitamin Revolution." The gist of the report was that there is a growing awareness within mainline circles of medical science and practice that vitamin and mineral supplements really *are* important for good health.

One of the individuals interviewed was Dr. Walter Willett, a Harvard epidemiologist (someone who tries to determine how diseases come about) who had been studying diet, supplements, and chronic disease. "Until quite recently," he said, "it was taught that everyone in this country gets enough vitamins through their diet and that taking supplements just creates expensive urine. I think we have proof that this isn't true. I think the scientific community has realized this is a very important area for research."[1]

Willett and his colleagues had just released the results of an eight-year study of more than 120,000 people that indicated that daily supplements of vitamin E of at least 100 International Units reduced the risk of heart disease by about 40 percent.

Of course, many health practitioners in this country who are more in tuned with the field of nutrition than those in mainline medicine had known and been teaching the importance of dietary supplements for years.

In his book *How to Get Well*, first published in 1974, Paavo Airola, Ph.D., N.D. (naturopathic physician), had this to say about vitamin and mineral supplements:

> Ideally, all vitamins, minerals, and other nutrients should be obtained from foods, without the addition of concentrated vitamins in pill or tablet form. This was possible 100 or 50 years ago, when all foods were grown on fertile soils, were unrefined and unprocessed, and contained all the nutrients nature intended them to contain. But today, when soils are depleted, when foods are loaded with residues of hundreds of toxic insecticides and other chemicals, and when the nutritional value of virtually all foods is drastically lowered by vitamin, protein, and enzyme destroying food-producing and food-processing practices . . . the addition of vitamins and

food supplements to the diet is of *vital importance*. Nutritionally inferior and poisoned foods of today cause many nutritional deficiencies, derangement in body chemistry, and lowered resistance to disease.[2]

Patrick Quillin, Ph.D., R.D. (Registered Dietician), wrote a book in 1987 in which he concurred with the conclusions of Dr. Airola. In *Healing Nutrients* he wrote: "Considering America's stressful lifestyle and ubiquitous pollution, our eat-on-the-run nutrient-depleted foods, our penchant for bizarre diets, and the possibility that many of us need greater-than-RDA levels of nutrients for optimal health, supplements are an essential part of the core nutrition program."[3]

The recommendation for daily supplements made by Dr. Quillin for average, healthy people include vitamins A, B-complex, C, D, and E, along with a complete mineral supplement (all the minerals are combined into one product). The label will tell you whether or not it is a complete mineral supplement. Follow the manufacturer's recommendations on the bottle as to when to take these supplements and how many.

Q. What if I want to develop health-promoting eating habits, but the rest of my family doesn't?

A. This is a good question. I just wish I could give a good answer. One woman in our local nutrition support group prepares two meals each evening, one for herself and the other for her husband, who doesn't wish to change. That's an answer. Not a fun one or an easy one, but an answer. If you truly wish to make changes in your own diet, you will often be faced with having to work very hard to do so.

If you've got kids, the opposition they will put up to dietary changes can be monumental. Work at it slowly and creatively. By preparing the best, tastiest, health-promoting meals you can, try to subtly seduce them toward better eating habits without a great deal of protest. It's a challenge, especially if your kids have become addicted to the fat, sugar, and salt in the standard American diet. But it can be done. In the process, set them a good example by your own eating habits. Be their model that they will look back upon in the future, even if they don't fully appreciate it today.

Another thing about eating habits and kids: Don't make eating poorly a sin. In other words, there *are* worse things kids could do. You want them to eat health-promoting foods, but their character and their values—these are even more important areas to shape. This certainly isn't meant to discourage you from trying to shape their eating habits and their experience of good health, but rather to encourage you to keep things in perspective.

As for you, it may be advantageous for you to join a nutrition support group to keep yourself motivated. Ask at health-food stores if they know of any in your locale. Another idea is to look up nutritionists, certified nutritional consultants, or naturopathic physicians in your yellow pages. Professionals like these may be your link to a support group. If all else fails, consider starting your own. All you need to get yourself started is a few extra copies of this book and some friends who would like to read, discuss, and share new meal ideas with each other. A couple of additional books you might wish to incorporate at some point might be:

▶ *A Cancer Battle Plan* (Piñon Press) by Anne and David Frähm

▶ *Fit for Life* (Warner Books) by Harvey and Marilyn Diamond

Q. My uncle and aunt lived on the farm, ate three huge meals containing meat and dairy products every day, smoked and drank, and both lived well into their nineties. In light of what you've been talking about in this book, how do you explain that?

A. Seems like we all know someone who appears to have violated all the rules of good health with impunity. Pure luck? Hardy genes? Who knows all the reasons why it happens?

The reality of life is that we're all very much alike, and yet biochemically unique at the same time. We will not all get colon cancer from a high-fat diet. We will not all get lung cancer from smoking. We will not all develop osteoporosis from a lifetime of consuming high-protein foods. But there are many who will. How do you know *you* won't be one of them? Is it really worth the gamble?

"Okay," you might be saying, "but no one in my family tree has ever had any of those things. I'm a product of one of those groups of people with hardy genes."

That's good, but are you aware of the fact that with cancer, for instance, 80 percent of the people who are being diagnosed these days have no trace of it in their family history? Genetic background does play some role in our individual health picture; however, our own diet and lifestyle are often even more significant.

And what of optimal, vibrant health right now—today? Are you really as healthy as you would like to be? Most of us would admit that we are not. Perhaps the problems you're dealing with on a regular basis are not life-threatening diseases, but headaches, allergies, constipation, recurrent sore throats, fatigue, yeast infections, sinus problems, stiff joints, or the like. Perhaps, like so many, you've resigned yourself to just live with it—to chalk it up as a normal part of life.

Up until my wife was diagnosed with widespread cancer, our family had given very little attention to studying our diet. We were your average American family, eating the standard American diet and suffering from those little things that seemed part of life. For instance, every six weeks or so during the winter months our kids would be at the doctor's office getting prescriptions for more antibiotics. It wasn't until our entrance into the world of nutrition, when all other means of fighting for Anne's life against cancer were exhausted, that we became aware of the importance of diet to health. Once we'd removed dairy products from our menu, our kids' problems with strep throat disappeared.

News is getting out. What we put into our mouths does affect our health. In the last dozen years or so some of the most sweeping changes Americans have been making in their lifestyles have had to do with food and eating habits. Many are experiencing a new sense of empowerment over the quality of their lives, not to mention lowering their risks for debilitating diseases and protecting themselves from escalating health-care costs.

Don't gamble with your health. The choice, of course, is yours. We'd love to have you join us.

NOTES

Chapter One: Take Charge

1. Gordon S. Tessler, *Lazy Person's Guide to Better Nutrition* (San Diego, CA: Better Health Publishers, 1984), page 2.
2. John A. McDougall, *McDougall's Medicine: A Challenging Second Opinion* (Piscataway, NJ: New Century Publishers, 1985), page 286.
3. Dean Ornish, *Dr. Dean Ornish's Program for Reversing Heart Disease* (New York: Ballantine Books, 1990), page 11.
4. McDougall, page 101.
5. John A. McDougall and Mary A. McDougall, *The McDougall Plan* (Piscataway, NJ: New Century Publishers, 1983), page 65.
6. Mike Samuels and Nancy Samuels, *The Well Adult* (New York: Summit Books, 1988), page 17.
7. Phil Gunby, "Battles Against Many Malignancies Lie Ahead as Federal 'War on Cancer' Enters Third Decade," *The Journal of the American Medical Association*, 8 April 1992, page 1891.

8. Samuels and Samuels, page 16.
9. Walter M. Bortz II, *We Live Too Short and Die Too Long* (New York: Bantam Books, 1991), page 6.
10. McDougall and McDougall, page 7.
11. William J. Kassler, "Testimony: Nutrition Education in the Undergraduate Medical Curriculum," *National Academy of Sciences*, 1 January 1985, page 121, as quoted by John Tepper Marlin with Domenick Bertelli, *The Catalogue of Healthy Food* (New York: Bantam Books, 1990), page 35.
12. Stuart M. Berger, *What Your Doctor Didn't Learn in Medical School* (New York: Morrow, 1988), page 19.
13. Ornish, page 12.
14. Charles B. Simone, *Cancer and Nutrition* (New York: McGraw-Hill, 1983), page xiv.
15. McDougall, *McDougall's Medicine*, page 101.

Chapter Three: Drink Pure Water

1. Joseph D. Weissman, *Choose to Live* (New York: Penguin Books, 1988), page 46.
2. Harper's Magazine, *What Counts: The Complete Harper's Index* (New York: Henry Holt and Co., 1991), page 145.
3. "Is Water Safe?" *U.S. News and World Report*, 29 July 1991, page 51.
4. "Your Guide to Produce," Wild Oats Community Market pamphlet, 1992.
5. "Is Water Safe?" page 53.
6. Gary Null, *Clearer, Cleaner, Safer, Greener* (New York: Villard Books, 1990), page 63.
7. "Is Water Safe?" page 53.
8. Null, page 57.
9. "Is Water Safe?" page 50.
10. William L. Fischer, *How to Fight Cancer and Win* (Canfield, OH: Fischer Publishing Corporation, 1987), page 234.
11. Allen E. Banik, *The Choice Is Clear* (Raytown, MO: Acres USA, n.d.), page 28.

12. Weissman, page 53.
13. Colin Ingram, *The Drinking Water Book* (Berkeley, CA: Ten Speed Press, 1991), page 24.
14. Weissman, page 52.
15. Andrew Weil, *Natural Health, Natural Medicine* (Boston: Houghton Mifflin, 1990), page 76.
16. "The Pollutants That Matter Most: Lead, Radon, Nitrate," *Consumer Reports*, January 1990, page 31.
17. Weil, page 76.
18. "Is Water Safe?" page 52.
19. "The Pollutants That Matter Most," page 31.
20. "The Pollutants That Matter Most," page 31.
21. "Is Water Safe?" page 51.
22. Ingram, page 18.
23. Ingram, pages 59, 60.
24. Weil, pages 76, 77.
25. Ingram, pages 63-66.
26. Ingram, pages 70, 71.
27. Banik, page 7.
28. Weil, page 78.
29. Ingram, from information scattered throughout the book.
30. Banik, page 10.
31. Harvey and Marilyn Diamond, *Living Health* (New York: Warner Books, 1987), page 92.
32. Weil, page 79.

Chapter Four: Cut Down on Fats and Oils

1. Udo Erasmus, *Fats and Oils* (Vancouver, Canada: Alive Books, 1986), page 299.
2. Erasmus, page 299.
3. Erasmus, page 201.
4. Dean Ornish, *Dr. Dean Ornish's Program for Reversing Heart Disease* (New York: Ballantine Books, 1990), page 264.
5. Ornish, page 264.
6. Erasmus, page 299.
7. David Reuben, *Everything You Always Wanted to Know*

About Nutrition (New York: Simon and Schuster, 1978), page 138.

8. Erasmus, page 101.
9. Andrew Weil, *Natural Health, Natural Medicine* (Boston: Houghton Mifflin, 1990), page 18.
10. Erasmus, pages 44, 135, 117.
11. Ornish, page 266.
12. Oliver Alabaster, as quoted by Neal D. Barnard, *The Power of Your Plate* (Summertown, TN: Book Publishing Co., 1990), page 56.

Chapter Five: Cut Down on Meat of All Kinds
1. Neal D. Barnard, *The Power of Your Plate* (Summertown, TN: Book Publishing Co., 1990), page 81.
2. John A. McDougall, *McDougall's Medicine: A Challenging Second Opinion* (Piscataway, NJ: New Century Publishers, 1985), page 108.
3. McDougall, page 99.
4. Barnard, page 15.
5. Udo Erasmus, *Fats and Oils* (Vancouver, Canada: Alive Books, 1986), page 246.
6. Maureen Salaman, *The Cancer Answer . . . Nutrition* (Menlo Park, CA: Statford Publishing, 1984), page 116.
7. Patrick Quillin, *Healing Nutrients* (Chicago: Contemporary Books, 1987), page 145.
8. McDougall, page 75.
9. McDougall, page 73.
10. Julian M. Whitaker and June Roth, *Reversing Health Risks* (New York: Putnam, 1988), page 79.
11. Michael F. Jacobson, Lisa Y. Lefferts, and Anne Wittee Garland, *Safe Food* (Los Angeles: Living Planet Press, 1991), page 93.
12. David Steinman, *Diet for a Poisoned Planet* (New York: Harmony Books, 1990), page 77.
13. John A. McDougall and Mary A. McDougall, *The McDougall Plan* (Piscataway, NJ: New Century Publishers, 1983), pages 51-52.

14. Jacobson, Lefferts, and Garland, page 93.
15. Steinman, page 80.
16. Joseph D. Weissman, *Choose to Live* (New York: Penguin Books, 1988), page 164.
17. Nathan Pritikin with Patrick M. McGrady, Jr., *The Pritikin Program for Diet and Exercise* (New York: Grosset and Dunlap, 1979), page 14.
18. Jacobson, Lefferts, and Garland, page 122.
19. "The Whole Story's Fishy," *Journal of Health and Healing*, Marjorie Baldwin, M.D., ed., as quoted by Kay Mirza, *Health Notes*, September 1992.
20. Mary Kerney Levenstein, *Everyday Cancer Risks and How to Avoid Them* (Garden City Park, NY: Avery Publishing Group, 1992), page 68.
21. Dean Ornish, *Dr. Dean Ornish's Program for Reversing Heart Disease* (New York: Ballantine Books, 1990), page 279.
22. Erasmus, pages 202-204.
23. Harvey and Marilyn Diamond, *Fit for Life* (New York: Warner Books, 1985), pages 71, 74.
24. McDougall, pages 73, 84.
25. Weissman, page 4.
26. Nathan Pritikin, as quoted in *Vegetarian Times* 43, page 22.
27. Frances Moore Lappe, *Diet for a Small Planet,* 10th anniversary edition (New York: Ballantine Books, 1982), pages 162, 172.
28. Whitaker and Roth, page 71.
29. Lappe, page 162.
30. David Reuben, *Everything You Always Wanted to Know About Nutrition* (New York: Simon and Schuster, 1978), page 185.
31. Quillin, pages 366, 367.

Chapter Six: Cut Down on All Dairy Products
1. Harvey and Marilyn Diamond, *Living Health* (New York: Warner Books, 1987), page 278.
2. Diamond, page 243.

3. John A. McDougall and Mary A. McDougall, *The McDougall Plan* (Piscataway, NJ: New Century Publishers, 1983), page 49.
4. Diamond, page 226.
5. McDougall and McDougall, page 50.
6. McDougall and McDougall, page 50.
7. Diamond, page 229.
8. McDougall and McDougall, page 54.
9. McDougall and McDougall, page 73.
10. Diamond, page 238.
11. McDougall and McDougall, page 52.
12. McDougall and McDougall, page 54.
13. McDougall and McDougall, page 51.
14. *The Nutrition Reporter*, vol. 3, no. 6, pages 1-2.
15. *The Nutrition Reporter*, page 2.
16. Diamond, page 248.
17. McDougall and McDougall, pages 70, 71.
18. Joseph D. Weissman, *Choose to Live* (New York: Penguin Books, 1988), page 78.
19. John A. McDougall, *McDougall's Medicine: A Challenging Second Opinion* (Piscataway, NJ: New Century Publishers, 1985), page 75.

Chapter Seven: Eat Lots of Raw, Organic Fruits and Vegetables

1. Ann Wigmore, *The Hippocrates Diet and Health Program* (Wayne, NJ: Avery Publishing Group, 1984), page 41.
2. Harvey and Marilyn Diamond, *Living Health* (New York: Warner Books, 1987), page 39.
3. Diamond, page 40.
4. Henry G. Bieler, *Food Is Your Best Medicine* (New York: Ballantine Books, 1965), page 202.
5. Norman W. Walker, *Colon Health: The Key to Vibrant Life* (Prescott, AZ: Norwalk Press, 1979), page 4.
6. Julian M. Whitaker and June Roth, *Reversing Health Risks* (New York: Putnam, 1988), page 133.

7. Richard O. Brennan, *Coronary? Cancer? God's Answer: Prevent It!* (Irvine, CA: Harvest House, 1979), page 128.
8. Wigmore, page 15.
9. Carlson Wade, *Helping Yourself with New Enzyme Catalyst Health Secrets* (West Nyack, NY: Parker Publishing Co., 1981), page 27.
10. Wigmore, pages 17-18.
11. Brennan, page 137.
12. Mary Ruth Swope with David A. Darbro, *Green Leaves of Barley* (Phoenix, AZ: Swope Enterprises, 1990), page 114.
13. John Tepper Marlin with Domenick Bertelli, *The Catalogue of Healthy Food* (New York: Bantam Books, 1990), page 61.
14. Michael F. Jacobson, Lisa Y. Lefferts, and Anne Witte Garland, *Safe Foods* (Los Angeles: Living Planet Press, 1991), page 45.
15. Jacobson, Lefferts, and Garland, page 48.
16. Mary Kerney Levenstein, *Everyday Cancer Risks and How to Avoid Them* (Garden City Park, NY: Avery Publishing Group, 1992), page 73.
17. Jacobson, Lefferts, and Garland, page 56.
18. Jacobson, Lefferts, and Garland, page 48.
19. Marlin, page 63.
20. Jacobson, Lefferts, and Garland, page 69.
21. Diamond, pages 29, 30.
22. Karen MacNeil, *The Book of Whole Foods* (New York: Vintage Books, 1981), page 165.

Chapter Eight: Build Cooked Meals Around Starches
1. Marilyn Diamond, *The American Vegetarian Cookbook* (New York: Warner Books, 1990), page 286.

Chapter Nine: Cut Back on Refined Sugars
1. Jane Brody, *Jane Brody's Nutrition Book* (New York: Bantam Books, 1981), page 119.
2. Marilyn Diamond, *The American Vegetarian Cookbook* (New York: Warner Books, 1990), page 327.

3. Brody, page 119.
4. Karen MacNeil, *The Book of Whole Foods: Nutrition and Cuisine* (New York: Vintage Books, 1981), pages 304-305.
5. Brody, page 121.
6. Brody, page 121.
7. Brody, page 121.
8. Brody, page 122.
9. Gordon S. Tessler, *Lazy Person's Guide to Better Nutrition* (San Diego, CA: Better Health Publishers, 1984), page 112.
10. MacNeil, page 312.
11. MacNeil, page 310.
12. MacNeil, page 305.
13. Brody, page 122.
14. Nancy Appleton, *Lick the Sugar Habit* (Garden City Park, NY: Avery Publishing Group, 1988), pages 42, 43.
15. David Reuben, *Everything You Always Wanted to Know About Nutrition* (New York: Simon and Schuster, 1978), page 206.
16. Tessler, page 186.
17. Tessler, page 89.
18. JoAnn Rachor, *Of These You May Freely Eat* (Sunfield, MI: Family Health Publications, 1986), page 83.
19. Diamond, page 327.
20. William G. Crook, *The Yeast Connection* (Jackson, TN: Professional Books, 1985), pages 17-26.
21. Appleton, pages 41-74.
22. Reuben, page 211.
23. Appleton, page 118.
24. John W. Rippon, as quoted by Crook, page 124.
25. Harvey and Marilyn Diamond, *Living Health* (New York: Warner Books, 1987), page 298.
26. Crook, page 124.

Chapter Ten: Cut Back on Salt
1. Patrick Quillin, *Healing Nutrients* (Chicago: Contemporary Books, 1987), page 96.

2. Robert A. Gleser, *The HealthMark Program for Life* (New York: McGraw-Hill, 1988), page 113.
3. Jane Brody, *Jane Brody's Nutrition Book* (New York: Bantam Books, 1981), page 203.
4. Brody, page 199.
5. Julian M. Whitaker and June Roth, *Reversing Health Risks* (New York: Putnam, 1988), page 84.
6. John A. McDougall, *McDougall's Medicine: A Challenging Second Opinion* (Piscataway, NJ: New Century Publishers, 1985), page 174.
7. McDougall, page 171.
8. Brody, page 207.
9. Neal D. Barnard, *The Power of Your Plate* (Summertown, TN: Book Publishing Co., 1990), page 25.
10. Gordon S. Tessler, *Lazy Person's Guide to Better Nutrition* (San Diego, CA: Better Health Publishers, 1984), page 79.
11. Annemarie Colbin, *Food and Healing* (New York: Ballantine Books, 1986), page 186.
12. Brody, page 204.
13. Brody, page 207.
14. Tessler, page 79.
15. Tessler, page 82.

Chapter Eleven: Choose Health-Promoting Snacks

1. Michael S. Lasky, *The Complete Junk Food Book* (New York: McGraw-Hill, 1977), page xvii.
2. Earl Mindell, *Earl Mindell's Safe Eating* (New York: Warner Books, 1987), page 118.
3. Nan Kathryn Fuchs, *The Nutrition Detective* (Los Angeles: Jeremy P. Tarcher, 1985), page 62.
4. Frances Sheridan Goulart, *The Carob Way to Health* (New York: Warner Books, 1982), page 3.
5. Goulart, pages 3,7.

Chapter Twelve: Cut Down on Tea and Coffee, Even Decaf

1. Jane Brody, *Jane Brody's Nutrition Book* (New York:

Bantam Books, 1981), page 235.

2. Donald M. Vickery, *Life Plan for Your Health* (Philippines: Addison-Wesley, 1984), page 155.

3. John A. McDougall, *McDougall's Medicine: A Challenging Second Opinion* (Piscataway, NJ: New Century Publishers, 1985), page 114.

4. Stuart M. Berger, *Dr. Berger's Immune Power Diet* (New York: New American Library, 1985), page 258.

5. McDougall, page 24.

6. John. A. McDougall and Mary A. McDougall, *The McDougall Plan* (Piscataway, NJ: New Century Publishers, 1983), page 175.

7. Brody, page 530.

8. Joseph D. Weissman, *Choose to Live* (New York: Penguin Books, 1988), pages 64, 65.

9. Mary Kerney Levenstein, *Everyday Cancer Risks and How to Avoid Them* (Garden City Park, NY: Avery Publishing Group, 1992), page 30.

10. Dr. Roland Griffiths, professor in the department of psychiatry and neuroscience at the Johns Hopkins University School of Medicine, quoted by Claudia Feldman, "Hooked on Caffeine," *Your Health* magazine, 29 December 1992, page 38.

11. Dean Ornish, *Dr. Dean Ornish's Program for Reversing Heart Disease* (New York: Ballantine Books, 1990), page 275.

12. Weissman, page 65.

13. Levenstein, page 32.

14. Dale and Kathy Martin, *Living Well* (Brentwood, TN: Wolgemuth and Hyatt, 1988), page 110.

Chapter Thirteen: Cut Back on Soft Drinks, Even Sugarless

1. Diane Campbell, *Step-by-Step to Natural Food* (Clearwater, FL: CC Publishers, 1979), page 157.

2. Mary Kerney Levenstein, *Everyday Cancer Risks and How to Avoid Them* (Garden City Park, NY: Avery

Publishing Group, 1992), page 30.

3. David Reuben, *Everything You Always Wanted to Know About Nutrition* (New York: Simon and Schuster, 1978), page 254.

4. Nan Kathryn Fuchs, *The Nutrition Detective* (Los Angeles: Jeremy P. Tarcher, 1985), page 2.

5. Fuchs, page 66.

6. Campbell, page 159.

7. Reuben, page 255.

8. Andrew Weil, *Natural Health, Natural Medicine* (Boston: Houghton Mifflin, 1990), page 49.

9. Joseph D. Weissman, *Choose to Live* (New York: Penguin Books, 1988), page 123.

10. Nathan Pritikin with Patrick M. McGrady, Jr., *The Pritikin Program for Diet and Exercise* (New York: Grosset and Dunlap, 1979), page 49.

11. Campbell, pages 2-3.

Chapter Fourteen: Cut Down on Alcohol

1. Allan Luks and Joseph Barbato, *You Are What You Drink* (New York: Stonesong Press, 1989), page 4.

2. Charles B. Simone, *Cancer and Nutrition* (New York: McGraw-Hill, 1983), page 106.

3. Luks and Barbato, page 34.

4. Luks and Barbato, page 59.

5. Nathan Pritikin with Patrick M. McGrady, Jr., *The Pritikin Program for Diet and Exercise* (New York: Grosset and Dunlap, 1979), page 46.

6. Luks and Barbato, page 61.

7. Frazer, as quoted by Luks and Barbato, page 61.

8. Nan Kathryn Fuchs, *The Nutrition Detective* (Los Angeles: Jeremy P. Tarcher, 1985), page 66.

9. Patrick Quillin, *Healing Nutrients* (Chicago: Contemporary Books, 1987), page 146.

10. Mary Kerney Levenstein, *Everyday Cancer Risks and How to Avoid Them* (Garden City Park, NY: Avery Publishing Group, 1992), page 24.

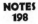

11. Quillin, page 113.
12. Luks and Barbato, page 88.
13. Annemarie Colbin, *Food and Healing* (New York: Ballantine Books, 1986), page 162.
14. Fuchs, page 66.
15. Simone, page 106.
16. Luks and Barbato, page 94.
17. Luks and Barbato, page 65.
18. Levenstein, page 23.
19. Joseph D. Weissman, *Choose to Live* (New York: Penguin Books, 1988), page 34.
20. Gleser, page 48.

Chapter Fifteen: Quit Smoking
1. Maury M. Breecher and Shirley Linde, *Healthy Homes in a Toxic World* (New York: John Wiley and Sons, 1992), page 34.
2. Mike Samuels and Nancy Samuels, *The Well Adult* (New York: Summit Books, 1988), page 136.
3. Harper's Magazine, *The Complete Harper's Index* (New York: Henry Holt and Co., 1991), page 149.
4. Samuels and Samuels, page 143.
5. Joseph D. Weissman, *Choose to Live* (New York: Penguin Books, 1988), page 31.
6. Samuels and Samuels, page 137.
7. From "Killing Us Softly," *Shape*, May 1993, page 17.
8. Harvey and Marilyn Diamond, *Living Health* (New York: Warner Books, 1987), pages 69-70.
9. Samuels and Samuels, page 141.
10. Holly Atkinson, *Women and Fatigue* (New York: Simon and Schuster, 1985), page 150.
11. Mary Kerney Levenstein, *Everyday Cancer Risks and How to Avoid Them* (Garden City Park, NY: Avery Publishing Group, 1992), page 250.
12. Diamond, page 75.
13. Levenstein, page 250.
14. Levenstein, page 250.

15. Weissman, page 32.
16. Weissman, page 32.
17. Levenstein, page 250.
18. Atkinson, page 155.
19. Levenstein, pages 252, 253.
20. Atkinson, page 159.

Chapter Sixteen: Exercise Regularly
1. Gordon S. Tessler, *Lazy Person's Guide to Better Nutrition* (San Diego, CA: Better Health Publishers, 1984), page 105.
2. Charles B. Simone, *Cancer and Nutrition* (New York: McGraw-Hill, 1983), page 159.
3. Kurt W. Donsbach with Morton Walker, *Metabolic Cancer Therapies* (Huntington Beach, CA: The International Institute of Natural Health Sciences, Inc., 1981), page 35.
4. Robert A. Gleser, *The HealthMark Program for Life* (New York: McGraw-Hill, 1988), page 142.
5. Simone, page 160.
6. Joseph D. Weissman, *Choose to Live* (New York: Penguin Books, 1988), page 90.
7. Gleser, page 143.
8. Gleser, page 145.
9. Tessler, page 110.
10. Dean Ornish, *Dr. Dean Ornish's Program for Reversing Heart Disease* (New York: Ballantine Books, 1990), page 336.
11. Dale and Kathy Martin, *Living Well* (Brentwood, TN: Wolgemuth and Hyatt, 1988), page 20.
12. Ornish, page 326.

Chapter Seventeen: Get Some Sun Regularly, But Carefully
1. Patrick Quillin, *Healing Nutrients* (Chicago: Contemporary Books, 1987), page 99.
2. Quillin, pages 311, 142.
3. Harvey and Marilyn Diamond, *Living Health* (New York:

Warner Books, 1987), page 175.

4. Dale and Kathy Martin, *Living Well* (Brentwood, TN: Wolgemuth and Hyatt, 1988), page 124.

5. Charles B. Simone, *Cancer and Nutrition* (New York: McGraw-Hill, 1983), page 48.

6. Karen Karvonen, "Toxic Tans: Why a Healthy Tan Hurts," *Women's Sports and Fitness*, July–August 1992, page 16.

7. Frances Munnings, "Sun Safety: Shedding Light on the Risks of Exposure," *The Physician and Sportsmedicine*, July 1991, page 100.

8. *Cancer Weekly*, 27 July 1992, page 10.

9. Sydney Hurwitz, as quoted by Alexandra Greely, "No Tan Is a Safe Tan: Depletion of the Ozone Layer Impairs Protective Screen Against Cancer-causing Radiation," *Nutrition Health Review*, Summer 1991, page 14.

10. *Cancer Weekly*, 27 July 1992, page 10.

11. Diamond, page 176.

12. Diamond, pages 176, 177.

13. Karvonen, page 16.

14. Simone, page 47.

15. Simone, page 49.

16. Dale and Kathy Martin, page 123.

17. James F. Balch and Phyllis A. Balch, *Prescription for Nutritional Healing* (Garden City Park, NY: Avery Publishing Group, 1990), page 289.

18. Michael J. Fransblau, "Suntan Parlors—A New Hazard to Health," *The Western Journal of Medicine*, February 1992, page 192.

19. Andrew Weil, *Natural Health, Natural Medicine* (Boston: Houghton Mifflin, 1990), page 178.

Chapter Eighteen: Breathe Clean Air

1. Harvey and Marilyn Diamond, *Living Health* (New York: Warner Books, 1987), page 59.

2. "Survey Finds 164 Million Americans at Risk from Air Pollution," *Colorado Springs Gazette Telegraph*, 30 April 1993.

3. Diamond, page 118.
4. Maury M. Breecher and Shirley Linde, *Healthy Homes in a Toxic World* (New York: John Wiley and Sons, 1992), page 32.
5. Mary Kerney Levenstein, *Everyday Cancer Risks and How to Avoid Them* (Garden City Park, NY: Avery Publishing Group, 1992), pages 117, 118.
6. David Steinman, *Diet for a Poisoned Planet* (New York: Harmony Books, 1990), page 245.
7. Levenstein, page 117.
8. Breecher and Linde, page 38.
9. Levenstein, page 187.
10. Breecher and Linde, page 34.
11. Levenstein, page 135.
12. Levenstein, page 117.
13. Levenstein, page 126.
14. Levenstein, pages 136, 137.

Chapter Nineteen: Effectively Deal with Negative Stress

1. James F. Balch and Phyllis A. Balch, *Prescription for Nutritional Healing* (Garden City Park, NY: Avery Publishing Group, 1990), page 297.
2. Gordon S. Tessler, *Lazy Person's Guide to Better Nutrition* (San Diego, CA: Better Health Publishers, 1984), page 100.
3. Richard O. Brennan with Helen Kooiman Hosier, *Coronary? Cancer? God's Answer: Prevent It!* (Irvine, CA: Harvest House, 1979), page 166.
4. Nancy Appleton, "Diet, Stress and the Immune System," *Towsend Letter for Doctors*, August/September 1992, pages 727, 728.
5. Mike Samuels and Nancy Samuels, *The Well Adult* (New York: Summit Books, 1988), page 51.
6. Tessler, page 102.
7. Ralph L. Woods, ed., *The World Treasure of Religious Quotations* (New York: Garland Books, 1966), pages 175, 61.